The Prepared Family Guide to Uncommon Diseases

This book is not meant to replace your family doctor or other health care worker. Consult your physician before attempting to diagnose and treat a disease.

Second Edition June 2012

Printed in USA

ISBN: 978-1-477-59385-1

Enola Gay
www.paratusfamiliablog.com
www.naturallycozy.com

Dedications

Enola Gay
To all of the Mothers, Grandmothers, Sisters and Aunts standing on the front lines ministering to their families and protecting their loved ones. Stand tall, arm yourselves and fight the good fight.

Grace Tome
To the aged women, that they teach the young women to be keepers at home, to care for their husbands and children. To all virtuous women, strength and honor are her clothing. She shall <u>rejoice</u> in time to come.

Maid Elizabeth
To my dad, Sir Knight, who gave me a love of all things medical. To Joe, my mentor, my friend.

Forward

This is a self-help book written by a person wanting to help themselves, who realized that this book could help others. Helping others is what people do best. The knowledge contained in this book is accurate and practical. The application of this knowledge by a caregiver requires accurate observations of the ill person, the time and the surroundings. If the observations of the caregiver do not match the information in the book, then think again and reassess the ill person.

Maurice F.P. Masar, MD, LMCC, FRSPH

NOTE: Dr. Masar's notes are included at the end of each chapter, in the "The Doctor Says..." section. Other comments by Dr. Masar are included in various sections, denoted by bold, italicized type.

From the Editor

This book began as a booklet that I intended to print out and put on my shelf so that I could reference its pages in the case of a medical emergency. But then, I wanted to give a copy to my parents and my brother and his family and my best friend, Dae. My eldest daughter, Maid Elizabeth, who had been helping with research needed a copy to take on her mission trip to the Philippines'. So did all of the other young ladies going with her. And then there were all of the families that we knew. They needed to have this information to take care of their families in a worst-case scenario situation.

And so, the booklet grew to be a full-fledged book. My modest desire to print out a copy or two became a burning desire to see it on as many shelves as possible. I wanted this information at my fingertips, if the worst should happen, and I wanted it available to every mother, daughter, grandmother and aunt who would be on the front lines of the battle, whether fighting a deadly epidemic or an inconvenient bought of chickenpox.

This book is not intended to replace your family doctor or other health professional. My mother, my daughter nor I have any medical expertise. We merely compiled facts and put them together in a format we found convenient and easily readable. We did our best to eliminate non-essential medical terminology and present nothing but the absolute bare essential information needed to identify, treat and contain a disease. Our goal was to equip people with the basic tools they needed to fight disease and win. We wanted the information to be as easily understood by a 12 year old girl and it was by her grandmother. *The Prepared Family guide to Uncommon Diseases* is the end result of our desire to equip ourselves and our loved ones with the knowledge to care for our families during a medical crisis.

Enola Gay
Paratus Familia

Sections

Section One
   Diseases

   Special Section

Section Two
   Recipes

Section Three
Treatment of Symptoms

Section Four
Baselines

Section Five
Shopping List

Section I

Diseases

Bubonic Plague

Description
What is it?

The term bubonic plague comes from the Greek word bubo, meaning "swollen gland". Swollen lymph nodes especially occur in the armpit and groin in persons suffering from bubonic plague. The bubonic plague refers to an infection that enters through the skin and travels through the lymphatic system. It is a flea-borne infection.

Signs/Symptoms
What does it look like?

Swollen lymph nodes are most commonly found in the armpits, groin or neck. Symptoms appear suddenly, usually 2-5 days after exposure to the bacteria. Symptoms include:
- Chills
- General malaise (not feeling well)
- High fever (102° Fahrenheit/39° Celsius)
- Seizures
- Painful lymph gland swelling found in groin, armpits or neck (most often at the site of the initial infection (bite or scratch).
- Pain may occur in the area before swelling is present.
- Heavy breathing
- Continuous blood vomiting
- Urination of blood
- Aching limbs
- Coughing

Additional symptoms may include:
- Extreme fatigue
- Gastrointestinal problems (tummy ache)
- Delirium
- Coma

Treatment
How do I care for my patient?

Treating the symptoms of the Bubonic Plague is recommended. Use a fever reducer (Tylenol, Ibuprofen, Aspirin) to control fever. Ice the inflamed lymph nodes to reduce swelling and offer pain relief. Antibiotics provide the only effective relief for the Bubonic Plague.

Recommended Antibiotics
- Streptomycin
- Tetracycline (especially Doxycycline)
- Ciprofloxacin

* The doctor's recommendation – The antibiotic of choice is Tetracycline of one form or another. If given IV (intravenous), should be 30 mg (milligrams) per kg (kilogram) of body weight per 24 hour period and given in divided doses. Or, it can be given orally at 500 mg (milligrams) every 6 hours for 5 days.

In humans, the bubonic plague kills about 2 out of every three infected patients *if left untreated.* Mortality is reduced to 1-15% if patient is treated.

Containment
How did I get it?
How do I keep it from spreading?

The Bubonic Plague is an infection that enters through the skin from the bite of infected fleas and small rodents. The plague is also known to spread to the lungs and become the disease know as the pneumonic plague. This form of the disease is highly communicable as the bacteria can be transmitted in droplets emitted when coughing or sneezing and also by physical contact with infected persons or with the flea bearing rodents that carry the plague.

Rodent control is a key component in containing a bubonic plague epidemic. When nursing a patient who's symptoms include coughing or sneezing, wearing personal protection equipment such as gloves and a face mask is indicated. Cleaning all surfaces in the sickroom with a chlorine bleach solution will keep the infection from spreading.

History

The Bubonic Plague was the cause of the Black Death that swept through Europe in the 14th century and killed an estimated 75 million people (30-60% of the European population).

The plague was used during the Second Sino-Japanese War as a biological weapon by the Imperial Japanese Army. It was testified that in 1941, plague-contaminated fleas were air-dropped on Changde. This operation caused epidemic outbreaks.

The Doctor says.....

Prompt and immediate treatment will reduce the mortality below 5%, where as without treatment the mortality is close to 100%. Some persons have a natural immunity and when supported by nutritious food and pulmonary exercises, do survive.

Chickenpox

Description
What is it?

Chickenpox is a highly contagious illness that begins with a skin rash mainly on the body and head and occurs most often in children. It is generally not life-threatening.

Signs/Symptoms
What does it look like?

Chickenpox is often identified by:

- Nausea
- Fever
- Headache
- Sore throat
- Ear aches (in one or both ears)
- Pressure in head or swollen face
- Malaise (not feeling well)
- Rash (generally beginning on stomach)
- Fever (from 100° F to 108° F)
- Anorexia (not eating well)
- Chickenpox lasts from 4 to 7 days

Chicken pox is generally more severe in adults than children and more severe in adult males than females. Chickenpox is rarely fatal.

NOTE: Pregnant women who have NOT had chickenpox should take extreme care not to be exposed to the virus during the first 28 weeks of pregnancy. Infection can severely affect the baby.

Treatment for Chickenpox mainly consists of easing the symptoms. There is no actual cure of the condition.

- Patients should cut their nails or wear gloves to prevent scratching and to minimize the risk of secondary infection
- Treat fever with a fever reducer (Tylenol, Ibuprofen – Aspirin is not recommended for children under the age of 16)
- Warm salt water gargle to relieve sore throat
- Warmed olive oil or garlic oil poured into ear canal to relieve earache
- Hot water bottle (covered in fleece) placed on ear to relieve earache
- Warm (not hot) oatmeal bath (just add a little oatmeal to water and stir), helps with itching
- Baking soda added to a warm (not hot) bath helps with itching.
- Vitamin E oil, Olive oil or honey can be used to sooth itching skin

Antibiotics are **not** indicated in the treatment of chickenpox.

Containment
How did I get it?
How do I keep it from spreading?

Chickenpox is contracted through close proximity to an infected person who is sneezing or coughing. The virus is also transmitted by physical contact with an infected person's lesions (the actual pox).

A person is contagious from a period lasting from three days prior to the onset of the rash, to four days after the onset of the rash. Once the pox have scabbed over, the person is no longer infectious.

History

Chickenpox is not related in any way to chickens. The name uses "chicken" in the sense of "weak" or "cowardly". The disease was given the name "chickenpox" because it is a "wimpier" version of smallpox.

The Doctor says....

Once a person has had chickenpox, the virus (varicella-zoster virus) resides in that person for the rest of their life. The virus stays in the nervous system, mainly the spinal cord. It can be activated by other diseases later in a person's life, or when their immune system is weakened by disease or an unhealthy life style. When the virus is activated it affects a nerve pathway so that vesicular lesions occur in a line on the chest or abdomen, and sometimes on the face and leading to the eye. Infection of the eye is particularly serious because it can result in blindness. Keeping the area clean is important. And comfort can be achieved by keeping ice packs on the affected area. There is now a herpes zoster immunization that is very effective. All adults should receive this immunization before the age of 60 years.

Cholera
Vibrio Cholerae

Description
What is it?

Cholera is an infection of the small intestine, sometimes referred to as Dysentery.

Signs/Symptoms
What does it look like?

Cholera is identified by:
- Profuse, painless, watery diarrhea
- Vomiting of clear fluids
- Diarrhea is describes as "rice water" and may have a fishy odor
- Untreated, the patient may produce 10-20 quarts (liters) of diarrhea a day, with fatal results

Treatment
How do I care for my patient?

Cholera must be aggressively treated within hours or it can result in life-threatening dehydration and electrolyte imbalances.

In most cases, cholera can be successfully treated with oral rehydration therapy (ORT) (see Oral Rehydration Therapy in the Recipes section), which is highly effective, safe and simple to do. In severe cases with significant dehydration, intravenous (I.V.) rehydration may be necessary. Ringer's lactate is the preferred solution for an I.V. drip.

Antibiotics will shorten the course of the disease and reduce the severity of the symptoms, however, people will recover without them, if sufficient hydration is maintained.

Recommended Antibiotics

- Doxycycline (typically used as first line of defense)
- Cotrimoxazole
- Erythromycin
- Tetracycline
- Chloramphenicol
- Furazolidone

* The Doctor's Recommendation – The antibiotics of choice are Tetracycline and Doxycycline. They are related and either one is effective.

Dose Schedule (Tetracycline/Doxycyline)

Adults:
500 mg (milligrams) given orally every 6 hours for 48 hours

Children:
250 mg (milligrams) every 6 hours for 48 hours

Furazolidone is also effective.

Dose Schedule (Furazolidone)

Adults:
100 mg (milligrams) given orally every 6 hours for 48 hours

Children:
50 mg (milligrams) every 6 hours for 48 hours

If people with cholera are treated quickly and properly, the mortality rate is less than 1%, however, if left untreated, the mortality rate jumps to 50-60%.

> **Containment**
> *How did I get it?*
> *How do I keep it from spreading?*

Cholera is typically transmitted by either contaminated food or water. The contamination is due to fecal (poop) material present in food or water, due to poor sanitation.

People infected with cholera often have diarrhea, and if this highly liquid stool contaminates water used by others, the disease may become an epidemic. The source of the contamination is typically other cholera sufferers when their untreated diarrheal discharge is allowed to get into waterways or into groundwater or drinking water supplies. Drinking infected water as well as eating foods washed in the water or eating shellfish living in the infected water can be a source of contamination. Cholera is rarely spread directly from person to person.

Prevention of cholera is simple if proper sanitation practices are followed. A cholera outbreak can be stopped by implementing the following safeguards:

- **Sterilization:** All materials that come in contact with either the infected patient or infected waste must be sterilized. Sterilization is accomplished by washing clothing, bedding, surfaces, etc. in hot water using chlorine bleach if possible. Hands should cleaned and disinfected with bleach or other antimicrobial agents (hot soap and water).
- **Sewage:** Antibacterial treatment of general sewage using chlorine bleach prevents inadvertently spreading the disease.
- **Sources:** Warnings about possible cholera outbreaks should be posted by any potentially contaminated waterways.
- **Directions for decontamination:** Boil (rolling boil) water for 1 minute or use 8 to 16 drops of bleach to 1 gallon of water. Double that amount for cloudy water.) This information should be posted as well.

History

Cholera became one of the most widespread and deadly diseases of the 19th century. Cholera is no longer considered a pressing health threat in Europe or North America due to filtering and chlorination of water supplies, but still heavily affects developing countries. In the past, people traveling in ships would hang a yellow quarantine flag if one or more of the crew members suffered from cholera. Passengers from boats that hung a yellow flag would not be allowed to disembark at any harbor for an extended period, typically 30 to 40 days. In modern international maritime signal flags, the quarantine flag is yellow and black.

The Doctor says....

Another type of oral rehydration is the "BRAT" diet. It consists of bananas, rice water, apple slices, and black or green tea. It is fed as often as possible to the ill person. Usually one episode of cholera produces immunity in the person.

Dengue
(Breakbone Fever, Dandy Fever)

Description
What is it?

This illness is sometimes confused with malaria because it is also caused by a virus that is spread by mosquitos. In recent years it has become much more common in many countries. It often occurs in epidemics (many people get it at the same time), usually during the hot, rainy season. A person can get dengue more than once, with repeat illnesses often being worse.

Signs/Symptoms
What does it look like?

- Sudden high fever with chills
- Sever body aches, headache, and sore throat
- Person feels very ill, weak, and miserable
- After 3 to 4 days person feels better for a few hours to 2 days
- The illness returns for 1 or 2 days, often with a rash that begins on hands and feet
- The rash then spreads to arms, legs, and finally the body (usually not the face)
- A severe form of dengue may cause bleeding into the skin (small dark spots), or dangerous bleeding inside the body

Treatment
How do I care for my patient?

No medicine cures dengue fever, but the illness goes away by itself in a few days.

Rest is important, as well as a lots of liquids. Acetaminophen (but **not** aspirin) will help with fever and pain.

In case of severe bleeding, treat for shock, if necessary.

Containment/Avoidance
How do I prevent or avoid it?

To prevent dengue, control mosquitos and protect against their bites, as described for malaria.

The Doctor says....

The most important things are keeping a person comfortable and hydrated. Because there are four different dengue viruses, a person has to develop immunity to each one, thus, a person can get dengue fever more than once.

Hantavirus

Description
What is it?

Hantavirus is a disease spread by rodents that presents similarly to the flu. Deer mice are a known Hantavirus carrier. The virus is in their urine and feces (poop), but it does not make the carrier animal sick. Humans become infected when they are exposed to contaminated dust from mice nests or droppings.

Signs/Symptoms
What does it look like?

Hantavirus symptoms are very much like flu symptoms, they include:
- Fever
- Chills
- Muscle aches

A person may feel better for a short time, then, within a day to two, develop shortness of breath. The disease worsens quickly and may lead to respiratory failure.

Other symptoms include:
- Dry cough
- Malaise (not feeling well)
- Headache
- Nausea
- Vomiting
- Rapid, shallow breathing
- Low blood pressure
- Hypoxia (low levels of oxygen, causing the skin to have a bluish color)

Treatment
How do I care for my patient?

An effective treatment for hantavirus infection involving the lungs is not yet available.

The treatment of Hantavirus consists of treating the symptoms. The best course of action is to take steps to not contract the disease in the first place.

Hantavirus is a serious infection. Even with aggressive treatment, more than half of the cases are fatal.

Containment
How did I get it?
How do I keep it from spreading?

The most effective way to combat Hantavirus is to take steps to prevent contraction of the disease.

| Transmission | Infected rodents shed the virus through urine, dropping and saliva. The virus is transmitted to humans by breathing contaminated dust or by contact with infected feces (poop), urine or nesting material. Infection can be transmitted through a bite by an infected animal, however, this is very rare.

Hantavirus cannot be transmitted from one person to another. It is not transmitted by farm animals, dogs or cats.

In the United States, deer mice (in the Northwest), cotton and rice rats (in the Southeast), and the white-footed mouse (in the Northeast) are the only known rodent carriers of Hantavirus. |
|---|---|
| Prevention | Keep your home clean. Clear out potential nesting sites and clean your kitchen.

When hiking and camping, pitch tents in areas where |

there are no rodent droppings.

Avoid rodent dens.

Drink disinfected water.

- When opening an unused cabin, shed or other building, open all the doors and windows, leave the building and allow the space to air out for 30 minutes.
- Return to the building and spray the surfaces, carpet and other areas with a disinfectant (Bleach solution: 1 ½ cups of bleach in 1 gallon water). Leave the buildings for another 30 minutes.
- Spray mouse nests and droppings with a 10% solution of chlorine bleach or similar disinfectant. Allow it to sit for 30 minutes. Using rubber gloves, place the materials in plastic bags. Seal the bags and throw them in the trash. Dispose of gloves and cleaning materials in the same way.
- Wash all potentially contaminated hard surfaces with a bleach or disinfectant solution. Avoid vacuuming until the area has been thoroughly decontaminated. Then, vacuum the first few times with plenty of ventilation. Surgical masks may provide some protection.

SEAL UP, TRAP UP, CLEAN UP
Seal up rodent entry holes or gaps with steel wool, lath metal or caulk. Trap rats and mice by using an appropriate trap. Clean up rodent food sources and nesting sites and take precautions when cleaning rodent-infested areas.

History

In 1993 there was an outbreak of fatal respiratory illness on an Indian reservation at the border of Utah, Colorado, New Mexico and Arizona. Researchers discovered that hantavirus caused the epidemic. Since that discovery, hantavirus disease has been reported in every western state and in many eastern states.

The Doctor Says.....

This is a very serious disease for which our immune system is not prepared. By the time a person is making antibodies, about 48 hours, their respiratory system is damaged and less oxygen is available to the body. Care of a person ill with this virus involves providing oxygen, respiratory therapy, hydration and pain relief with acetaminophen. The caregiver must take precautions not to breath in any respiratory droplets from the ill person, and to wash their hands after touching the ill person.

Head Lice

Description
What is it?

Head lice are tiny insects that live on the scalp. They can be spread by close contact with other people. Head lice infect hair on the head. They are easiest to see on the neck and over the ears. Head lice can survive up to 30 days on a human. Their eggs can live for more than 2 weeks.

Signs/Symptoms
What does it look like?

Tiny eggs on the hair look like flakes of dandruff, however, unlike dandruff, they do not flake off the scalp – they stay put. Other symptoms include:

- Intense itching of the scalp
- Small red bumps on the scalp, neck and shoulders (bumps may become crusty and ooze)
- Tiny white specks (eggs, also known as nits) on the bottom of each hair. They are very difficult to remove

Treatment
How do I care for my patient?

Lice can be killed quickly and safely with mayonnaise. Put a handful (or several handfuls) of mayonnaise on hair and cover all of the hair. Make sure to get behind the ears and down the neck a little. You can cover this with a plastic shower cap to keep the mayonnaise from dripping. Leave the hair covered for two hours to smother the lice and developed eggs. Remove and dispose of the shower cap, wash hands thoroughly and shampoo hair. It may take two or more shampoos to get the hair clean.

You can use Vaseline if you don't have any mayonnaise. To remove the Vaseline from the hair, saturate the hair in baby oil, rub in thoroughly and squeeze out as much as you can. Wash the hair as many as three times with Dawn dish soap and hot water, leaving the dish soap on for a few minutes each time to allow it to work.

Another option is a natural lice shampoo:

5 tsp. Pure Olive Oil (or Pure Coconut Oil)
5 drops Tea Tree Essential Oil
5 drops Rosemary Essential Oil
5 drops Lavender Essential Oil
5 drops Peppermint Essential Oil
5 drops Eucalyptus Essential Oil

Add a small amount of regular shampoo to the mixture and massage through hair. Leave on hair for an hour under a towel or tight-fitting shower cap to prevent drips. Rinse and shampoo the hair.

(The olive oil or coconut oil kill lice by dissolving their exoskeletons – other oils will not have the same effect)

NOTE: 1) The respiration of a baby or child under 5 can be slowed down or even stopped if peppermint oil or eucalyptus oil is close enough for the baby to breathe. 2) High blood pressure may be elevated by peppermint essential oil. 3) Peppermint or rosemary may be harmful during pregnancy. In any of these cases, just use the recipe without the oil that may be harmful in your case.

After treatment you must remove the eggs:
- You can remove the eggs with a nit comb. Before doing this, rub olive oil in the hair or run the metal comb through beeswax. This helps make the nits easier to remove
- Metal combs with very fine teeth are stronger and more effective than plastic nit combs. These metal combs are easier to find in pet stores or online than in pharmacies
- Removing eggs may prevent the lice from returning if the shampoos are ineffective
- Treat children and adults with lice promptly and thoroughly.

- Wash all clothes and bed linens in hot water with detergent. This also helps prevent head lice from spreading to others during the short period when head lice can survive off the human body
- Repeat combing for nits in 7 to 10 days

Containment
How did I get it?
How do I keep it from spreading?

Head lice spreads easily. You can get head lice when you come in close contact with a person who has lice, or by touching their clothing or bedding. Head lice are more common in close, overcrowded living conditions.

Controlling the spread of head lice requires treating the lice and properly sanitizing clothing and bedding that has come into contact with an infected person.

The Doctor Says.....

Lice are usually found where personal hygiene has been neglected or prevented, such as in the elderly, infants, refugees and prisoners. Even a daily plain water bath is effective in controlling them. And, washing one's clothes and bedding regularly is important.

Malaria

Malaria is an infection of the blood that causes chills and high fever.
Malaria is spread by mosquitos. The mosquito sucks up the malaria
parasites in the blood of an infected person and injects them into the next
person it bites. People with HIV are twice as likely to catch malaria.

Signs/Symptoms
What does it look like?

- The typical attack has 3 stages:
  1. It begins with chills – and often headache. The person shivers
     or shakes for 15 minutes to an hour.
  2. Chills are followed by fever, often 104° F or more. The
     person is weak, flushed (red skin), and at times delirious (not
     in his right mind). The fever lasts several hours or days.
  3. Finally the person begins to sweat, and his temperature goes
     down. After an attack, the person feels weak, but may feel
     more or less OK.
- Usually malaria causes fevers every 2 or 3 days (depending on the
  kind of malaria), but in the beginning it may cause fever daily.
  Also, the fever pattern may not be regular or typical. For this
  reason anyone who suffers from unexplained fevers should have
  his blood tested for malaria
- Chronic malaria often causes an enlarged spleen and anemia
- In young children, anemia and paleness can begin within a day or
  two. In children with malaria affecting the brain (cerebral malaria),
  seizures (fits) may be followed by periods of unconsciousness.
  Also, the palms may show a blue gray color, and breathing may be
  rapid and deep. (**Note:** Children who have not been breast fed are
  more likely to get malaria)

If you suspect malaria or have repeated fevers, if possible go to a health center for a blood test.

In areas where malaria is common, treat any unexplained high fever as malaria. Take a malaria medicine.

Recommended Medications: (can be used in two ways – some only for Treatment and some only for Prevention and others for both)
- Artemisinin
- Chloroquine (Doctor's Choice)
- Chloroquine Phosphate
- Chloroquine Sulfate
- Quinine
- Mefloquine
- Pyrimethamine with sulfadoxine
- Primaquine

If you get better with the medicine, but after several days the fevers start again, you may need another medicine.

Containment/Avoidance
How did I get it?
How do I keep it from spreading?

Malaria occurs more often during hot, rainy seasons. If everyone cooperates, it can be controlled. All these control measures should be practiced at once.

1. **Avoid mosquitos:** Sleep where there are not mosquitos or underneath a bed net treated with insecticide or under a sheet. Cover the baby's cradle with treated mosquito netting or a thin cloth.
2. **Cooperate with medical workers:** Tell them if anyone in the family has had fevers and let them take blood for testing.

3. **If you suspect malaria, get treatment quickly:** After you have been treated, mosquitos that bite you will not pass malaria on to others.
4. **Destroy mosquitos and their young:** Mosquitos breed in water that is not flowing. Clear ponds, pits, old cans, or broken posts that collect water. Raise mosquito-eating fish in ponds or lakes.
5. Malaria can also be prevented, or its effects greatly reduced, by taking anti-malaria medicines on a regular schedule.

The Doctor says....

Of all the drugs listed, Chloroquine is the most helpful and is usually available in the drug store. It can be used as a preventative.
Preventative Dosage

Adults:
500 mg (milligrams) orally once a week, starting one week before entering a malaria zone. Continue the dosage for one week after leaving the malaria zone.

Children:
250 mg (milligrams) orally once a week, starting one week before entering a malaria zone. Continue the dosage for one week after leaving the malaria zone.

Acute Dosage (if you have malaria)

Adults:
1 Gram orally, followed in 6 hours by 500 mg (milligrams) orally, then 500 mg (milligrams) orally for 2 days.

Children:
500 mg (milligrams) orally, then in 6 hours 250 mg (milligrams) orally, and the next day 250 mg (milligrams) orally.

Measles
Morbillivirus

Description
What is it?

Measles (sometimes known as English Measles) is an infection of the respiratory system caused by the measles virus. Measles is highly contagious – 90% of people without immunity sharing living space with an infected person will catch it.

Signs/Symptoms
What does it look like?

Symptoms of measles include:
- Fevers up to 104° F
- Cough
- Runny nose
- Conjunctivitis (red eyes)
- Spots inside mouth (often not present)

Two to four days after initial symptoms an infected person may develop a rash, starting on the head before spreading to cover most of the body. This rash if often itchy and appears as a "stain" over the body that begins as a red color changing to dark brown before disappearing after about eight days.

Complications can include:
- Diarrhea
- Pneumonia
- Encephalitis (swelling of the brain)
- Ear infection

Treatment
How do I care for my patient?

There is no specific treatment for measles. Most patients will recover with rest and supportive treatments (treating the symptoms).

- Treat fevers with Tylenol, Ibuprofen or Aspirin (aspirin is not recommended for children under 16)
- Tea bags soaked in warm water and used as a compress on eyes will relieve conjunctivitis
- If diarrhea becomes severe, offer ORT (oral rehydration therapy)
- Bronchodilator for cough (Primatene Mist (available only through 12/11), Albuterol)

Containment
How did I get it?
How do I keep it from spreading?

Measles is spread through respiration (contact with fluids from an infected person's nose and mouth, either by physical contact or being sneezed upon). The infection has an incubation period of 14 days and the ability to pass on the infection lasts from 2 – 4 days prior to symptoms until 2 – 5 days following the onset of the rash.

Precautions to take when caring for a measles patient:
- PPE (personal protection equipment – which includes gloves and a surgical mask)
- Clean infected surfaces with a chlorine bleach solution
- Quarantine of the infected person will help stop the spread of the disease

History

The Antonine Plague, 165-180 AD, also known as the Plague of Galen, who described it, was probably smallpox or measles. The disease

42

decimated the Roman army. Measles is an endemic disease, meaning that it has been continually present in a community and many people develop a resistance. In populations that have not been exposed to measles, exposure to a new disease can be devastating.

The Doctor says....

Measles was brought to the new world by the incoming European Settlers. It killed as much as 60-70% of the Indian Tribes on initial contact. Those that survived developed immunity to the disease, and their children were born with an increased level of resistance to the disease.

Mumps

Description
What is it?

Mumps is a viral disease causing painful swelling of the salivary glands. Painful testicular swelling and rash may also occur. The disease is generally limited, running its course with no specific treatment apart from controlling the symptoms.

Signs/Symptoms
What does it look like?

The symptoms of Mumps include:
- Painful swelling of the salivary glands (sometimes one gland, but more commonly both glands are affected)
- Fever
- Headache
- Painful swelling of the testicles (30% of males past puberty experience this symptom)

Other symptoms that can occur:
- Dry mouth
- Sore face
- Earaches
- Loss of voice

Treatment
How do I care for my patient?

There is no specific course of treatment for the mumps. In an effort to provide comfort, the symptoms must be treated.
- Swelling may be relieved by the application of intermittent ice and heat to the affected area (either neck or testicular area). Twenty minutes of ice followed by a twenty minute resting period followed by twenty minutes of heat.

- Fever reducers such as Tylenol or Ibuprofen (which also help control pain) to control pain and fever.
- Warm salt water gargles to reduce throat pain.
- Soft foods and extra fluids are recommended

Containment
How did I get it?
How do I keep it from spreading?

Mumps is a contagious disease that is spread from one person to another through contact with respiratory secretions such as saliva from an infected person or infected droplets from an infected person sneezing or coughing. The infection can also survive on surfaces and then spread after contact in a similar manner. A person with mumps is contagious from 6 days before the onset of symptoms until 9 days after symptoms start.

To contain the spread of the disease:
- Quarantine patient in own room
- Wear a surgical mask when entering sick room
- Clean infected surfaces with a bleach/water solution
- Wash hands thoroughly after contact with infected person
- Wash linens of infected person with hot water and bleach

History

Mumps is first described in the writings of the ancient Greek physician Hippocrates, who wrote during the 5th century B.C.
Epidemics of the mumps occurred during the 18th and 19th centuries. The outbreaks occurred worldwide, often in close quarters, such as military barracks, boarding schools, ships at sea and prisons. In World War I, mumps was the leading cause of French troops missing active duty.

When mumps occurs in the late teens and twenties, it tends to affect one or both testicles of the male person, and, rarely the ovaries of the female person. This usually results in that organ becoming sterile. Cooling the testicles with ice can prevent some damage. That is, the testicles can produce sperm, but at a lower number. This may require some special techniques later on when the male person wants to father a child.

Pneumonia
Community acquired

Description
What is it?

Pneumonia is an inflammatory condition of the lung. Often the air sacks (alveoli) in the lungs are filled with fluid, thus reducing the air capacity. There are numerous causes of pneumonia including bacteria, viruses, fungi and parasites. Typical symptoms include cough, chest pain, fever and difficulty breathing. For our purposes, we are going to examine community-acquired pneumonia (CAP).

Signs/Symptoms
What does it look like?

Community-acquired pneumonia is infectious pneumonia in a person who has not recently been hospitalized. CAP is the most common type of pneumonia. The signs and symptoms of pneumonia include:
- Cough producing greenish or yellow phlegm
- High fever accompanied by shaking chills
- Shortness of breath
- Chest pain
- Sharp or stabbing pain during deep breaths or coughs
- May cough up blood
- Headaches
- Sweaty and clammy skin

Other possible symptoms:
- Loss of appetite
- Fatigue
- Blueness of skin
- Nausea/vomiting
- Mood swings

- Joint pain or muscle aches
- In the elderly, may cause delirium (confusion)

You may be able to predict if your patient has pneumonia by examining the following chart:

Findings
- Fever over (100° F)
- Pulse over 100 beats/minute
- Rawls/crackles (does their chest crackle when they breath)
- Decreased breath sounds
- *Absence* of asthma

Diagnosis based on number of findings
- 5 findings – 84% to 91% probability
- 4 findings – 58% to 85%
- 3 findings – 35% to 51%
- 2 findings – 14% to 24%
- 1 findings – 5% to 9%
- 0 findings – 2% to 3%

Treatment
How do I care for my patient?

Typically, oral antibiotics, rest, fluids and home care are sufficient for complete recovery. As with most other illnesses, treatment of the symptoms is indicated.

- Treat fever with Tylenol, Ibuprofen or Aspirin (aspirin is not recommended for children under the age of 16)
- Resting while "propped" up will help relieve shortness of breath and make it easier to breath.
- Warm lemon juice with honey helps relieve coughing and soothes the throat.
- Antibiotics are indicated for Community-acquired Pneumonia. The antibiotics listed are used for treating CAP:

- Amoxicillin
- Erythromycin
- Azithromycin
- Doxycycline

The duration of treatment with antibiotics has traditionally been seven to ten days, however there is increasing evidence that short courses (three to five days) are as effective.

Containment
How did I get it?
How do I keep it from spreading?

Community-acquired pneumonia enters the lungs when airborne droplets are inhaled, but can also reach the lungs through the bloodstream when there is an infection in another part of the body. Standard "infection control" practices are advised to halt the spread of the disease.

Infection Control
- Wash hands in hot, soapy water
- Wear a surgical mask while attending an infected patient
- Cover mouth when coughing or sneezing
- Wash infected surfaces with a bleach/water solution
- Sterilize linens by washing in hot, soapy water with bleach

---

History

The symptoms of pneumonia were first described by Hippocrates (c. 460–370 BC), however he referred to pneumonia as a disease "named by the ancients". Maimonides (1138-1404 AD) observed "The basic symptoms which occur in pneumonia and which are never lacking are as follows: acute fever, sticking pain in the side, short rapid breaths, serrated pulse and cough".

The Doctor says....

Community Acquired Pneumonia does not mean that the bacteria or virus is of some type that will make everyone ill. Instead, it means that the person who developed pneumonia, did so because of some weakness in

their immune system. Perhaps stress, over work, fatigue, smoking and the causal agent can be found in most everybody in the community even though they are not ill. Because it affects the lungs, which are vital for a person's survival, especially in the elderly and the very young, respiratory therapy is very important. This amounts to regular deep breathing exercises and coughing up phlegm. Antibiotics help the body to resist the infecting agent, and must be used in conjunction with respiratory therapy.

The most useful antibiotics are Tetracycline, Amoxicillin and Ciprofloxin. There is a pneumonia immunization available, and every person over 30 years of age should have this immunization protection.

Pertussis
Whooping Cough

Description
What is it?

Pertussis, also know as whooping cough is a highly contagious bacterial disease. Symptoms are initially mild and then develop into severe coughing fits, which produce the namesake high-pitched "whoop" sound in infected babies and children when they inhale air after coughing.

Signs/Symptoms
What does it look like?

The signs and symptoms of pertussis begin with:
(*one to two weeks in duration*):
- Mild respiratory symptoms
- Mild coughing
- Sneezing
- Runny nose

Followed by:
(*two to eights weeks in duration*):
- Coughing
- Whooping after coughing
- Vomiting after coughing
  Secondary symptoms may include:
  - Urinary incontinence
  - Post-cough fainting

The disease culminates with decreased coughing, both in frequency and severity, and a cessation of vomiting. This is the convalescent stage, lasting one to two weeks.

Treatment
How do I care for my patient?

Treatment for pertussis consists of treating symptoms and administering antibiotics.

Effective treatment of the cough associated with this disease have not yet been developed, although herbal treatments and vitamin C in the form of sodium ascorbate have been said to greatly decrease the severity of the cough caused by pertussis.

Antibiotics, while shortening the infectious period, do not generally alter the outcome of the infection. When antibiotic treatment is introduced in the early stages of the disease, symptoms may be less severe.

Antibiotics used for treatment of Pertussis:
- Erythromycin
- Azithromycin
- Clarithromycin
- Trimethoprim-sulfamethoxazole

The duration of treatment with antibiotics is 10 – 14 days.

Containment
How did I get it?
How do I keep it from spreading?

Pertussis enters the system when infected airborne droplets are inhaled. Standard infection control measures will help stop the disease from spreading.

Infection Control
- Wash hands in hot, soapy water
- Wear a surgical mask while attending an infected patient
- Cover mouth when coughing or sneezing
- Wash infected surfaces with a bleach water solution
- Sterilize linens by washing in hot, soapy water with bleach

54

There is an immunization for whooping cough that most children receive. However, this immunization decreases as a person grows older. By age 60, a person is no longer protected against the cause, Bordetella pertussis bacteria, and can be infected again. This time the elderly person does not have the typical whooping cough, but may have a frequent dry cough. However, the bacteria are spread in the cough droplets to infants, children and adults resulting in severe breathing problems for those who have not been immunized, and who have other health problems. Elderly persons should be re-immunized against whooping cough. While antibiotics do help reduce the severity of the symptoms, they also prevent spread of the disease by the cough droplets.

Radiation Poisoning

Description
What is it?

Radiation poisoning, also referred to as radiation sickness, occurs when someone is exposed to large enough levels of radiation to create damage to the body. Radiation poisoning rarely occurs outside of nuclear industrial operations. It could affect the general public during nuclear-weapons testing or in an attack using nuclear weapons.

Radiation poisoning, radiation sickness or radiation toxicity is a constellation of health effect which occur within several months of exposure to high amounts of ionizing radiation. The term generally refers to acute problems rather than ones that develop after a prolonged period.

Signs/Symptoms
What does it look like?

The speed of onset of symptoms is directly related to radiation exposure, with greater doses resulting in a shorter delay of symptoms onset. Mild radiation poisoning (radiation doses as low as 35 rad) presents in this manner:

- Nausea
- Vomiting
- Headaches
- Fatigue
- Fever
- Short periods of skin reddening

Cutaneous radiation syndrome (CRS) is the skin symptoms of radiation exposure. Within a few hours after irradiation:

- Itching
- Reddening
- Blistering
- Ulceration (open sore)

Gastrointestinal symptoms (typical with exposure doses of 600-1000 rad), usually seen within 1 to 2 hours:

- Nausea
- Vomiting
- Loss of appetite
- Abdominal pain

Neurovascular symptoms (typical with exposure doses greater than 1000 rad):

- Dizziness
- Headache
- Decreased level of consciousness
- Absence of vomiting

Treatment
How do I care for my patient?

There is no cure for radiation poisoning, however, prompt treatment can lessen the effects.

Particle Removal
One of the first and most basic treatments for radiation poisoning is the thorough removal of any particles on the skin and clothing. To do this, all clothing should be removed and disposed of. This should get rid of about 90 percent of the radiation contamination. Washing with soap and warm water helps removed any other particles that may still be clinging to the skin. It is important to do this immediately after exposure, as active particles on skin and clothing can continue to poison.

Potassium Iodide (K1)
Potassium iodide is a common treatment option for radiation poisoning. Potassium iodide collects in the thyroid. It takes up space that radioactive iodine would occupy. Without room to stay in the thyroid, the radioactive iodine is sent out of the thyroid and excreted with urine. Take Potassium Iodide orally either before or after exposure, although it works best if taken before exposure.

Dosage:
- Adult – (1) 130 mg. tablet once a day for 10 days
- Children – (1) 62 mg. tablet once a day for 10 days

Iodine can also be obtained by rubbing iodine on the skin, particularly on the belly and allowing it to be absorbed.

The Doctor Says: K1 can be used in older persons. K1 won't hurt them and it is used only for a short time. K1 can also be used by persons on Thyroid medication for hypothyroidism without harm.

Prussian Blue
Prussian blue may also be used to treat radiation poisoning. Prussian blue binds with radioactive particles in the body. It binds with two other types of radioactive elements called thallium and cesium. When taken directly after exposure, Prussian blue is able to remove many of the radioactive particles before the cells can absorb them. Once attached to the radioactive particles, the Prussian blue exits the body in the feces (poop), taking along the particles.

Prussian blue is safe for most adults, including pregnant women, and children (2 –12 years). Dosing for infants (ages 0 –2 years) has not been determined yet. Women who are breast feeding their babies should stop breast feeding if they think they are contaminated with radioactive materials.

Dosage:
- Adult – (1) 500 mg. tablet 3 times daily for a minimum of 30 days
- Children – ½ of an adult dose

Prussian blue has been included in the SNS (Strategic National Stockpile).

The Doctor Says: I don't know anything about using Prussian Blue for the treatment of radiation poisoning. It is a chemical composed of iron and cyanide and is a deep blue powder with a distinctive odor. It is non-toxic. It combines with thallium and cesium, so that when these metals are radioactive as produced by a nuclear explosion, it prevents their absorption

into the blood stream by removing them from the intestine. It is usually given in 500 mg per day doses for 7 days. Dosages as high as 3 times daily are not going to cause any harm.

Containment
How did I get it?
How do I keep it from spreading?

The best prevention for radiation sickness is to minimize exposure. Radiation poisoning cannot be transmitted via airborne droplets. It can only be spread via direct contact or radioactive fallout. Remove any contaminated clothing or equipment that has come in contact with radiation and put them in a double plastic bag labeled RADIOACTIVE. Bury the bag in three feet of earth.

The Doctor Says....

Because a person cannot see "radioactivity" it is scary. Yet, keeping your head and using your common sense will keep you from being harmed. I grew up down wind from the Hanford Nuclear Research Center in Washington. Yes, the dust was radioactive, but we did not collect enough of it in our bodies to harm us. Later in my life, I was in Norway after the Chernobyl nuclear disaster. The radioactive clouds went to the northwest into the Scandinavian countries. My group was picking up samples of weeds, grass and other foliage. My group had been assembled rapidly and we deployed without our normal field rations. So I contacted a cooking school, and they supplied us daily with freshly baked bread and delicious reindeer stew. After several days of eating this, we managed to get a Geiger counter to test for radiation. The stew was radioactive. We were monitored for several years after this, but nothing bad happened to us. Probably the most important thing to remember is to get out of the downwind area from a nuclear or radioactive disaster. A person needs to move so that they are not breathing in the dust or collecting it on their clothes or allowing it to contaminate their food.

Rubella
German Measles

<table>
<tr><td>Description
What is it?</td></tr>
</table>

Rubella, commonly know as German Measles is a viral infection. The name "rubella" is derived from the Latin, meaning little red. This disease is often mild and attacks often pass unnoticed. The disease can last one to three days. Children recover more quickly than adults. Rubella can be serious in pregnant women, particularly during the first 20 weeks of pregnancy.

<table>
<tr><td>Signs/Symptoms
What does it look like?</td></tr>
</table>

Rubella (German Measles) causes symptoms that are similar to the flu. The primary symptom of rubella is the appearance of a rash on the face, which spreads to the trunk and limbs and usually fades after three days. The facial rash usually clears as it spreads to other parts of the body.

Other symptoms include:
- Low grade fever (rarely rises above 100.4° F)
- Swollen glands (can persist for up to a week)
- Joint pain
- Headache
- Conjunctivitis (red or goopy eyes)

<table>
<tr><td>Treatment
How do I care for my patient?</td></tr>
</table>

There is no specific treatment for Rubella other than treating the symptoms.

- Low grade fever does not require treatment
- Swollen glands can be relieved with hot/cold packs
- Joint pain can be lessened with an OTC (over the counter) pain reliever (no aspirin for children under 16 years of age)
- Headache can be treated with an OTC pain reliever
- Conjunctivitis can be treated with moist towels (compress) soaked in tea or eye bright (herb). The water should be warm to provide maximum relief

Containment
How did I get it?
How do I keep it from spreading?

Rubella is transmitted via airborne droplet emission from the upper respiratory tract of infected people. The virus may also be present in the urine, feces (poop) and on the skin of infected persons.

Standard "infection control" measures will help stop the spread of the disease:
Infection Control
- Wash hands in hot, soapy water
- Wear a surgical mask while attending an infected patient
- Cover mouth when coughing or sneezing
- Wash infected surfaces with a bleach water solution
- Sterilize linens by washing in hot, soapy water with bleach

History
Rubella is also known as German measles because the disease was first described by German physicians in the mid-eighteenth century.

The Doctor Says....

This is a very mild illness. The only very important thing to remember is to keep females who may be pregnant away from the infected person for at least a week after the rash has disappeared. The virus causes very severe defects in an unborn child.

Scarlet Fever

Description
What is it?

Scarlet fever is a disease caused by Streptococcus pyogenes. Once a major cause of death it is now effectively treated with antibiotics.

Signs/Symptoms
What does it look like?

Scarlet Fever is characterized by:
- Sore throat
- Fever (at or above 101° F)
- Swollen glands in neck
- Tonsils may be covered with a whitish coating or appear red, swollen and dotted with whitish or yellowish specks of puss
- Bright red tongue with a "strawberry appearance"
- Characteristic rash, which is fine, red and rough-textured; it is blanched upon pressure. The rash appears 12 to 48 hours after the fever. The rash usually appears first on the neck and face, often leaving a clear unaffected area around the mouth. It spreads to the chest and back and then to the rest of the body. It worsens in the skin folds.

The rash begins to fade three to four days after onset and peeling then begins.

A person with Scarlet fever may have:
- Chills
- Body aches
- Nausea
- Vomiting
- Loss of appetite

Treatment for Scarlet fever consists of treating the symptoms and administering antibiotics.

The infection itself is usually cured with a 10 day course of antibiotics, but it may take a few weeks for tonsils and swollen glands to return to normal. Patients should no longer be infectious after taking antibiotics for 24 hours.

The Doctor Recommends:
Penicillin is the antibiotic of choice. A single dose of 1.2 million units IM (intramuscular) for adults and 600,000 units IM (intramuscular) for children suffices. When penicillin is contraindicated (person is allergic) then use erythromycin with a dose of 500 mg (milligrams) orally twice daily for 10 days for adults and 250 mg (milligrams) orally twice daily for children.

Containment
How did I get it?
How do I keep it from spreading?

Scarlet fever is transmitted via airborne droplet emission from the upper respiratory tract of infected persons.

Standard "infection control" measures will help stop the spread of the disease:

Infection Control
- Wash hands in hot, soapy water
- Wear a surgical mask while attending an infected patient
- Cover mouth when coughing or sneezing
- Wash infected surfaces with a bleach/water solution
- Sterilize linens by washing in hot, soapy water with bleach

The bacteria is spread by droplets or touch, so good infection control measures are important to stop the spread. The bright redness of the skin of a person with scarlet fever is sometimes frightening. The red skin is not infective, only the lesions in the tonsils are infective.

Smallpox

Description
What is it?

Smallpox is a serious, contagious, and sometimes fatal infectious disease. There are two forms of smallpox, Variola Major, the severe and most common form of smallpox and Variola Minor, the less common, less severe form of smallpox.

The last naturally occurring case of smallpox in the world was in Somalia in 1977. After the disease was eliminated from the world, routine vaccination against smallpox among the general public was stopped because it was no longer necessary for prevention.

Signs/Symptoms
What does it look like?

Symptoms of smallpox include:
- Fever (at least 101° F)
- Muscle pain
- Headache
- Nausea
- Vomiting
- Backache
- Rash

Incubation Period (Duration: 7 to 17 days) *Not contagious*	Exposure to the virus is followed by an incubation period during which people do not have any symptoms and may feel fine. This incubation period averages about 12 to 14 days but can range from 7 to 17 days. During this time, people are not contagious.

Initial Symptoms (Duration: 2 to 4 days) *Sometimes Contagious*	The first symptoms of smallpox include fever, malaise (not feeling well), head and body aches and sometimes vomiting. The fever is usually high, in the range of 101° to 104° F. At this time, people are usually too sick to carry on their normal activities.
Early Rash (Duration: about 4 days) *Most contagious*	A rash emerges first as small red spots on the tongue and in the mouth. These spots develop into sores that break open and spread large amounts of the virus into the mouth and throat. At this time, the person becomes most contagious. Around the time the sores in the mouth break down, a rash appears on the skin, starting on the face and spreading to the arms and legs and then to the hands and feet. Usually the rash spreads to all parts of the body within 24 hours. As the rash appears, the fever usually falls and the person may start to feel better. By the third day of the rash, the rash becomes raised bumps. By the fourth day, the bumps fill with a thick, opaque fluid and often have a depression in the center that looks like a bellybutton. (This is a major distinguishing characteristic of smallpox.) Fever often will rise again at this time and remain high until scabs form over the bumps.
Pustular Rash (Duration: about 5 days) *Contagious*	The bumps become pustules – sharply raised, usually round and firm to the touch as if there's a small bound object under the skin. People often say the bumps feel like BB pellets embedded in the skin.

Pustules and Scabs **(Duration: about 5 days)** *Contagious*	The Pustules begin to form a crust and then scab. By the end of the second week after the rash appears, most of the sores have scabbed over.
Resolving Scabs **(Duration: about 6 days)** *Contagious*	The scabs begin to fall off, leaving marks on the skin that eventually become pitted scars. Most scabs will have fallen off three weeks after the rash appears. The person is contagious to others until all of the scabs have fallen off.
Scabs resolved *Not contagious*	Scabs have fallen off. Person is no longer contagious.

Treatment
How do I care for my patient?

There is no cure for smallpox. After symptoms start, treatment consists of supportive medical care, including giving the person fluids to prevent dehydration and medicines to control pain and fever.

- Treat fever with Ibuprofen or Tylenol
- Administer ORT (oral rehydration therapy) to prevent dehydration

Containment
How did I get it?
How do I keep it from spreading?

Generally, direct and fairly prolonged face-to-face contact is required to spread smallpox from one person to another. Smallpox also can be spread through direct contact with infected bodily fluids or contaminated objects such as bedding or clothing. Rarely, smallpox has been spread by virus carried in the air in enclosed settings such as buildings, buses and trains. Smallpox is not known to be transmitted by insects or animals.

In temperate areas, the number of smallpox infections are highest during the winter and spring. In tropical areas, seasonal variations are less evident and the disease is present throughout the year.

Standard infection control measures will help stop the spread of the disease:

Infection Control
- Wash hands in hot, soapy water
- Wear a surgical mask while attending an infected patient
- Cover mouth when coughing or sneezing
- Wash infected surfaces with a bleach water solution
- Sterilize linens by washing in hot, soapy water with bleach

History

In 1796 Edward Jenner, a doctor in Berkeley, Gloucestershire, rural England, discovered that immunity to smallpox could be produced by inoculating a person with material from a cowpox lesion. Cowpox is a poxvirus in the same family as variola. Jenner called the material used for inoculation vaccine, from the root word vacca, which is Latin for cow. The procedure was much safer than variolation, and did not involve a risk of smallpox transmission. Vaccination to prevent smallpox was soon practiced all over the world.

The Doctor Says.....

Smallpox was once well known to all physicians, but since 1977, no one has really seen a case and the subject is not taught in medical schools anymore. My last case was in the 1960's in Algeria in North Africa. It was a teenage boy who had the typical lesions. He survived and had very few disfiguring pits on his skin. Good sanitation and wearing a mask will protect the caregiver.

Starvation

Description
What is it?

Starvation is the result of a severe or total lack of nutrients needed for maintaining life. It is a continued and extreme deprivation of food resulting in morbid effects.

Signs/Symptoms
What does it look like?

Starved adults may lose as much as 50% of their normal body weight. Characteristic symptoms of starvation include:
- Chronic diarrhea
- Anemia
- Reduction in muscle mass resulting in weakness
- Lowered body temperature (extreme sensitivity to cold)
- Decreased ability to digest food because of lack of digestive acid production
- Irritability and difficulty with metal concentration
- Immune deficiency
- Swelling from fluid under the skin (protein deficiency)

Complete starvation in adults leads to death within eight to 12 weeks. In the final stages of starvations, adults experience a variety of other symptoms including:
- Hallucinations
- Convulsions
- Severe muscle pain
- Disturbances in hearth rhythm

In children, starvation symptoms include:
- Growth retardation
- Mental retardation

Other symptoms in both children and adults include:

- Anemia (low iron resulting in tiredness and pale skin)
- Swelling of the legs (due to lower levels of protein in the blood)
- Loss of resistance to infection
- Poor wound healing
- Progressive weakness
- Difficulty swallowing

Treatment	
How do I care for my patient?	

The treatment of starvation depends on the severity of the condition.

Moderate Starvation (loss of less than 20% body weight)	Treatment for moderate starvation (loss of less than 20% body weight and where there is no diarrhea) consists of any available food. A person with moderate starvation may take in 4,000 calories a day (or more) and gain up to 4 pounds a week. Begin treatment with a clear liquid diet, quickly progressing to a healthy, balanced diet.
Severe Starvation (loss of up to 50% body weight)	If the patient is enfeebled, and especially if diarrhea is severe, extreme caution is necessary in treatment. Unsuitable food may result in death. Introduction of frequent, small feedings of nutritious, easily digestible foods are needed until the patient's digestive tract has had a chance to recover. Treat with a liquid diet, slowly progressing to a diet of soft foods over the course of three days. **First, Second and Third Day of Treatment:** *First Day:* <ul><li>Frequent offerings of a mixture of Starvation Fluids</li></ul>Second Day: <ul><li>Gruels made from local grains</li><li>Toast or bread</li></ul>*Third Day:* <ul><li>A regular, full, well-balanced meal</li></ul>

Shock is very likely to result in cases of severe starvation. No attempt to give food or water by mouth should be made until the shock has been treated. Keeping your patient at rest, in a warm bed is of the greatest importance in treating starvation. If your patient has trouble swallowing, a dry mouth and difficulty urinating, you must treat them for thirst before giving them soft or solid foods.

Starvation Fluids

½ C dried skim milk (prepared with water)
1/3 C edible oil
¼ C Sugar

Mix together adding ground up vitamins if available. Feed frequently throughout the first 24 hours of treatment.

The Doctor Says.....

Remember that it is not necessary to give lots of food right away. Small amounts at intervals will bring the patient back to health. Tiny infants are a special case. They require someone 24 hours a day to nurture them and provide whatever liquid or liquefied food is available, and only in very small amounts.

Tetanus

<table>
<tr><td>Description
What is it?</td></tr>
</table>

Tetanus is a serious bacterial disease that affects the nervous system. Tetanus results when a germ that lives in the feces (poop) of animals or people enters the body through a wound. The disease causes painful muscle contractions, especially in the neck and jaw (thus, the term "lockjaw"). Tetanus can interfere with your ability to breath.

<table>
<tr><td>Signs/Symptoms
What does it look like?</td></tr>
</table>

The incubation period of tetanus can be from 8 days to several months. The further the injury site is from the central nervous system, the longer the incubation period. The shorter the incubation period, the more severe the symptoms.

There are four different forms of tetanus:

Generalized Tetanus	This is the most common type of tetanus. It represents about 80% of tetanus cases. Generalized tetanus symptoms are: • Lockjaw • Facial spasms • Stiffness of the neck • Difficulty in swallowing • Rigid pectoral (upper arm) and calf muscles Other signs may include: • Fever • Sweating • High blood pressure • Rapid heart rate • Drooling

Neonatal Tetanus	This is a form of generalized tetanus that occurs in newborns. It usually occurs through infection of the unhealed umbilical stump, particularly when the umbilical cord has been cut with a non-sterile instrument. It appears 3 to 10 days after birth. The child begins to cry continuously and is unable to suck. It is very important to start treating tetanus at the first sign. If you suspect tetanus (or if a newborn child cries continuously or stops nursing), conduct this test: TEST OF KNEE REFLEXES • With the leg hanging freely, tap the knee with a knuckle just below the kneecap. • If the leg jumps just a little bit, the reaction is normal. • If the leg jumps high, this indicates a serious illness like tetanus (or perhaps meningitis or poisoning with certain medicines or rat poison). • This test is especially useful when you suspect tetanus in a newborn baby.
Local Tetanus	Local tetanus is an uncommon form of the disease. With local tetanus, patients have repeated contraction of the muscle group nearest to the injury. The contraction of muscles may persist for weeks before gradually lessening. Local tetanus is often milder than generalized tetanus, however, it may precede the onset of generalized tetanus.
Cephalic Tetanus	Cephalic tetanus is an uncommon form of the disease, occasionally occurring with an ear infection, or following injuries to the head. There is generally involvement of the facial nerves.

There are currently no blood tests that can diagnose tetanus. Tetanus is typically diagnosed by symptoms and ruling out other diseases with similar symptoms. One diagnostic method is called the "spatula test". This test consists of touching the back of the throat with a sterile, soft-tipped instrument and observing the effect. If the patient has an involuntary clamping of the jaw (biting down on the "spatula"), it is indicative of a positive result for tetanus. If the patient gags in an attempt to expel the "spatula", most likely tetanus is not present.

Treatment
How do I care for my patient?

Puncture wounds and other deep cuts, animal bites or very dirty wounds put you at risk for a tetanus infection. Proper care must be taken when dealing with a wound with possible tetanus infection.

Wound care:
- Clean the wound. After the bleeding has stopped, rinse the wound thoroughly with clean, running water (saline solution is preferable, if available). Clean the area around the wound with soap and a washcloth. Clean out any embedded debris.
- After cleaning the wound, apply a layer of antibiotic ointment such as Neosporin or Bag Balm.
- Cover the wound. Bandaging the wound will keep it clean and discourage bacteria. Keep the wound covered until a scab forms.
- Change the wound dressing every day or whenever the wound becomes dirty or wet. This will help prevent infection.

If infection has occurred, it must be treated with antibiotics and antitoxin (tetanus immune globulin), if available. If you can get it, inject 5,000 units of Human Immune Globulin or 40,000 to 50,000 units of Tetanus Antitoxin. Human Immune Globulin has less risk of severe allergic reaction, but may be more expensive and harder to obtain.

Effective antibiotics include:
- Metronidazole (most effective)
- Penicillin (1 million units of procaine penicillin at once and repeat every 12 hours)
- Clindamycin
- Erythromycin

Other comforting measures are:
- Muscle relaxers
- Bed rest with a non-stimulating environment (dim light, no noise, comfortable temperature)

Containment
How did I get it?
How do I keep it from spreading?

Tetanus cannot be transmitted from one person to another. The bacteria is harbored in the ground. Infection begins when the bacteria enter the body through an injury or a wound. Many people associate tetanus with rusty nails. This is only true if the nail is dirty as well as rusty. It is the dirt on the nail, not the rust, that carries the risk for tetanus.

Vaccination is the surest protection against tetanus. Both children and adults should be vaccinated. For complete protection, the vaccination should be repeated once every 10 years. Vaccinating women against tetanus each time they are pregnant will prevent tetanus in newborn infants.

The Doctor Says......

Cleaning the wound is the most important activity for preventing a tetanus infection. The second most important item is to get the tetanus immunization every 10 years.

Tuberculosis

Description	
What is it?	

"TB" is short for tuberculosis. Historically, TB was known as "Consumption". The TB disease is caused by a bacteria that usually attacks the lungs but can attack any part of the body, such as the kidney, spine and brain.

Signs/Symptoms	
What does it look like?	

Not everyone infected with TB becomes sick. Because of this, there are two types of TB conditions that exist: Latent TB infection and Active TB disease.

Latent TB Infection (not contagious)	TB can live in your body without making you sick. If you have contracted the TB bacteria, but show no signs or symptoms, you have latent TB. Most people who breathe in TB bacteria and become infected have the immune system to fight the bacteria and keep them from growing. People with latent TB do not feel sick and do not have any symptoms. People with latent TB are not infectious and cannot spread TB bacteria to others. If a persons immune system is compromised, the TB bacteria can become active and multiply, causing the person to get sick with active TB disease.
TB Disease (contagious)	TB bacteria becomes active if the immune system can't stop them from growing. Symptoms may include: • Bad cough that lasts 3 weeks or longer • Pain in the chest • Coughing up blood or sputum • Weakness or fatigue

	- Weight loss - No appetite - Chills - Fever - Sweating at night

Treatment
How do I treat my patient?

No treatment is required for latent TB. Aggressive treatment is required for active TB disease. Treatment of active TB will always involve a combination of many drugs (usually four). The most commonly used drugs include:

- Isoniazid
- Rifampin
- Pyrazinamide
- Ethambutol

Other drugs that may be used to treat TB include:

- Amikacin
- Ethionamide
- Moxifloxacin
- Para-aminosalicylic acid
- Streptomycin

TB treatment requires taking four different pills at different times of the day for 6 months (or longer). Not taking the appropriate medications for the suggested duration may make the infection more difficult to treat as the bacteria may become resistant to treatment.

Containment
How did I get it?
How do I keep it from spreading?

It is by far easier to stop the spread of TB than it is to treat the active disease. TB is spread through the air from one person to another. The TB bacteria are put into the air when a person with active TB disease of the lungs or throat coughs, sneezes, or speaks. People nearby may breathe in the bacteria and become infected.

When dealing with a patient with active TB, standard infection control measures are encouraged.

Infection Control
- Wash hands in hot, soapy water
- Wear a surgical mask while attending an infected patient
- Cover mouth when coughing or sneezing
- Wash infected surfaces with a bleach water solution
- Sterilize linens by washing in hot, soapy water with bleach

The Doctor Says....

Because there is a resurgence of TB throughout the world, it must be guarded against. A cough that seems to last too long should be investigated. Giving antibiotics without consideration that the case may be TB may cause the TB infection to become resistant.

Typhoid Fever

Description
What is it?

Typhoid fever, also known as typhoid, is a common worldwide illness, transmitted by the ingestion of food or water contaminated with the feces (poop) of an infected person. The impact of this disease falls sharply with modern sanitation techniques.

Signs/Symptoms
What does it look like?

Typhoid fever is characterized by a slowly progressive fever, (as high as 104° F), profuse sweating and gastrointestinitis (tummy ache). In some cases a rash of flat, rose-colored spots may appear.

Untreated typhoid fever is divided into four stages, each lasting approximately one week.

Week 1
- Slowly rising temperature
- Bradycardia (slow heartbeat)
- Malaise (exhaustion)
- Headache
- Cough
  Other possible symptoms
  - Bloody nose
  - Abdominal pain

Week 2
- Bedridden
- High fever (104 degrees)
- Bradycardia (slow heartbeat)
- Slow, thready pulse

- Delirium
- Rose spots on lower chest and abdomen (in 1/3 of patients)
- Rhonchi lung sounds (Rhonchi are sounds that resemble snoring. They occur when air is blocked or becomes rough through the large airways) lung sounds are best heard with a stethoscope.
- Abdomen is distended (bloated) and painful
- Diarrhea, 6 to 8 stools (poops) a day, green, with a characteristic smell, with the consistency of pea soup.
- Constipation could be present instead of diarrhea

Week 3
- Neuropsychiatric symptoms (severe delirium – known as the typhoid state) with picking at bedclothes or imaginary objects.
- Dehydration

Week 4
- Convalescence

Treatment
How do I care for my patient?

Treatment for Typhoid Fever consists of treating the symptoms and administering antibiotics.

- Oral Rehydration Therapy is indicated for the treatment of diarrhea
- Tylenol, Ibuprofen or Aspirin (not for children under the age of 16) for the fever

Antibiotics commonly used to treat Typhoid Fever:
- Ampicillin
- Chloramphenicol
- Trimethoprim-sulfamethoxazole
- Amoxicillin
- Ciprofloxacin

In resistant populations:
- Azithromycin

When untreated, typhoid fever persists for three weeks to a month. Death occurs in between 10% and 30% of untreated cases.

Containment
How did I get it?
How do I keep it from spreading?

Flying insects feeding on feces (poop) occasionally transfer the bacteria through poor hygiene habits and public sanitation conditions.

Typhoid can only spread in environments where human feces or urine are able to come into contact with food or drinking water. Careful food preparation and washing of hands are crucial to preventing typhoid.

- Outhouse or human waste disposal **must** be at least 150 feet from any water source
- Treat contaminated water with chlorine bleach (16 drops of bleach to 1 gallon of water – let settle for 10 minutes)
- Wash hands with hot water and soap before preparing or handling food
- Do not consume contaminated food
- Keep flies from landing on food

Standard "infection control" measures will help stop the spread of the disease:

Infection Control
- Wash hands in hot, soapy water
- Wash infected surfaces with a bleach water solution
- Be particularly mindful of handling human waste from the infected person

Sterilize linens and soiled clothing by washing in hot, soapy water with bleach.

History

Around 430-424 BC, a devastating plague, which some believe to have been typhoid fever, killed one third of the population of Athens, including their leader Pericles.

Some historians believe that in the English colony of Jamestown, Virginia, typhoid fever killed more than 6000 settlers between 1607 and 1624. During the American Civil War, 81,360 Union soldiers died of typhoid or dysentery.

The Doctor Says.....

Salmonella typhi is the bacteria responsible for typhoid fever, but the major cause is unhygienic health practices. Food and a person's hands contaminated by fecal material are the two most common causes. Contaminated well or spring water is also a significant cause. Lastly, the control of flies will diminish the spread of typhoid fever.

Typhus

Description
What is it?

Typhus is any of several similar diseases caused by Rickettsia. It comes from the Greek typhos, meaning smoky or hazy, describing the state of mind of those affected with typhus. The cause of typhus is a parasite that cannot survive for long outside of living cells. Typhus should not be confused with typhoid fever, as the diseases are unrelated. Multiple diseases include the word "typhus" in their description. Types include:

Condition	Arthropod	Notes
Epidemic Typhus	Lice on Human	When the term "typhus" is used without qualification, this is usually the condition meant.
Murine Typhus or "endemic typhus"	Fleas on rats	
Scrub Typhus	Harvest mites on humans or rodents	Scrub typhus is currently not classified in the typhus group, but in the closely related spotted fever group
Queensland tick typhus or Australian tick typhus (or spotted fever)	Ticks	

Murine Typhus:

- Abdominal pain
- Backache
- Dull red rash that begins on the middle of the body and spreads
- Extremely high fever (105°-106° F)
- Hacking, dry cough
- Headaches
- Joint pain
- Nausea
- Vomiting

Epidemic Typhus

- Chills
- Bad cough
- Delirium
- High fever (104° F)
- Joint pain
- Low blood pressure
- Rashes
- Sensitivity to light
- Severe headaches
- Severe muscle pain
- Stupor

Treatment
How do I care for my patient?

Without treatment, this disease can be fatal. Prompt treatment with antibiotics cures every patient.

Indicated antibiotics:

- Doxycycline
- Tetracycline
- Chloramphenicol (less common)

Containment
How did I get it?
How do I keep it from spreading?

Murine typhus occurs in the southeastern and southern United States, often during the summer and fall. Risk factors for murine typhus include:
- Exposure to rat fleas or rat feces (poop)
- Exposure to other animals such as cats, opossums, raccoons, and skunks

Endemic typhus is usually seen in areas where hygiene is poor and the temperature is cold. Endemic typhus is sometimes called "jail fever".

To prevent typhus, you must avoid areas where you might encounter rat fleas or lice. Good sanitation and hygiene are vital. Take measures to reduce the rat population.

When an infection has been found, you must take measures to rid persons of lice (which cause the disease). These measures include:
- Bathing
- Boiling clothes
- Avoiding infested clothes or bed linens for at least 5 days (lice will die without feeding on blood)
- Wash hair with lice shampoo and use metal nit comb to rid scalp of eggs.

History

Typhus was common in prisons (and in crowded conditions where ice spread easily). It often occurs when prisoners are frequently huddled together in dark, filthy rooms. During WWII the U.S. military controlled typhus by spraying soldiers with DDT.

The prevention of typhus is mainly through the use of DDT and good hygienic practices for the body and one's clothes. The antibiotics, Tetracycline and Chloramphenicol do not kill the infecting agents, but rather stop them from multiplying, allowing the body time to mount an immune system response. Because this takes time, nursing care is most important.

Special Section

Good Home Treatment of Influenza

A practical guide to home care of mild to severely ill patients that relies on a simple common sense approach.

By Grattan Woodson, M.D., FACP
Author of the Bird Flu Preparedness Planner and the Bird Flu Manual

This excerpt may be copied and distributed in part or in whole without a licensing fee as long as it is properly referenced as below.

Grattan Woodson, MD, FACP
August 29, 2006

Grattan Woodson, MD, FACP
2801 North Decatur Rd., Suite 375
Decatur, GA USA 30033

This special section is an excerpt from Dr. Woodson's booklet entitled "Good Home Treatment of Influenza". The content was so exceptional and complete, I couldn't see fit to change a word. *Enola Gay*

The Great Bird Flu Pandemic

It is in the nature of all influenza pandemics to cause widespread illness and death. As during seasonal flu, the vast majority of those sick with pandemic flu will be treated at home by their family members and friends. This guide was written for people taking care of mildly to severely ill influenza patients in their home who have no formal medical training.

A pandemic will last between 12 to 18 months and over that time about half the people on earth will become sick. Most will be mild to moderately ill, but some will be very sick. This guide will help you take care of these people at home using simple methods and do not rely on prescription drugs, medical equipment or medical training.

At times during a severe pandemic, hospitals could become full of sick and dying patients, running out of space for new patients. Access to doctors may become limited. Medical supplies and drugs could be in short supply. If these things happens, people like you with no prior formal medical training may find yourself caring for terribly ill loved ones and friends, who under normal circumstances would be treated by the doctor in the hospital. Home care, while not up to the standards of hospital care, can still be very effective. The simple methods found in this guide are those that have the power to keep patients from dying from the common, preventable causes of death from influenza such as dehydration.

What is "good home care" for the flu?

Good home care is nine parts common sense and one part simple medical practice. Taking care of someone with flu will be a familiar task for those who have nursed family members back to health in the past as it relies on simple common treatments and techniques.

The Flu Treatment Kit

Providing good care to family members and friends sick with influenza is a task that will be easier with a good supply of select over-the-counter medications, some medical equipment, and a few items from the grocery or hardware store. These items form the basis of the Flu Treatment Kit (FTK).

The Flu Treatment Kit (items for one person)
Grocery Store Items

- Table salt: 1 lb (for making Oral Rehydration Solution, gargle and nasal wash)
- Table sugar: 10 lbs (for making Oral Rehydration Solution)
- Baking soda: 6 oz. (for making Oral Rehydration Solution and nasal wash)
- Household bleach, unscented: 2 gal. (for purifying water and cleaning contaminated items)
- Caffeine containing tea, bags or dry loose: 1 lb (for treatment of respiratory symptoms)
- Two 8 oz. Plastic baby bottles with rubber nipples *1 (for administering Oral Rehydration Solution to severely ill)
- Two 16 oz. plastic squeeze bottle with swivel nozzles (for administering Oral Rehydration Solution to the ill)
- Two kitchen measuring cups with 500cc (two cup) capacity (for measuring lots of things)
- One set of kitchen measuring spoons 1/2tsp up to 1Tbsp. (for making oral solution and dosing)
- Fifty soda straws (for administering fluids)
- One composition-style notebook (for keeping a medical record on the patient)
- Teakettle *2 (for steam therapy)

FTK Items found at the drug store

- Petroleum jelly 4 oz. *3 (for lubrication of tubes, suppositories, and skin treatment and protection)
- Cocoa butter, pure, 2oz. *4 (for making suppositories and skin treatment and protection)
- An accurate bathroom scale (for weighing)
- Two electronic thermometers *5 (to measure temperature)
- Automatic blood pressure monitor (to measure blood pressure)
- Humidifier (for increasing the relative humidity of the air breathed by the patient)
- Pill cutter (to make it easier to reduce the dose of medications if desired)

- 1 box of Latex gloves #100, (to help reduce contamination and spread of the virus and bacteria)

Non-Prescription drugs

- Ibuprofen 200mg (Motrin) # 100 tablets (for treatment of flu symptoms)
- Diphenhydramine (Benadryl) 25mg capsules #100 (for treatment of flu symptoms)
- Robitussin DM Cough Syrup or its generic equivalent (12 oz) (for treatment of cough)
- Acetaminophen 500mg (Tylenol) #100 tablets (for treatment of flu symptoms)
- Loperamide 2mg #100 tablets (for diarrhea and abdominal cramps)
- Meclizine 25mg #100 tablets (for nausea and vomiting)

FTK Items found at the hardware store

- N-95 masks #20 (2 boxes) (to reduce diseases spread to and from the patient)
- 50 gallon sturdy plastic garbage container with top (used to store clean water for drinking)

Abbreviations: 1b = pound, oz = ounce, gal = gallon, # = number, cc = cubic centimeters, tsp = teaspoon, tbsp. = tablespoon, mg = milligrams, hrs = hours

Useful home care medical procedures

Home caregivers will be better able to evaluate and treat their patients by learning a few simple medical procedures. This includes taking the patient's vital signs: pulse, blood pressure, temperature, weight, and respiratory rate. Blood pressure is easily measured using an automated blood pressure monitor. Follow the instructions that come with the device to learn how to use it. The pulse is provided on the blood pressure monitor readout. It can be measured directly by feeling the pulse at the wrist and counting how many beats pass in 15 seconds and multiplying by 4. Temperature is measured directly with a digital thermometer. The patient's weight is measured on a scale in the standard manner and is best taken with the patient lightly dressed without shoes and around the same time each day. Watching for and counting the breaths taken over a 15 second period and multiplying the count by 4 provides the patient's respiratory rate. "Practice makes perfect" applies to learning the perfecting these skills.

How flu is passed person-to-person

Don't worry about contacting the flu because it will contact you. Almost everyone is vulnerable to a new flu strain. There is nothing unusual about this; influenza pandemics are a regularly occurring event with one happening on average 3 times each century. Humankind is well prepared to suffer these pandemics and bounce back as we have many times in the past. Pandemic influenza is so infectious; it is quite natural for the majority of the population to contract the virus before it is brought under control by our body's immune systems. About half of the people who contract the virus will have typical flu symptoms, and the other half will have very few, if any, symptoms. So while everyone is susceptible to a new strain, for reasons that we do not understand at present, only half the people exposed get sick.

Another reason pandemic flu is passed so easily from person to person is that people infected with the virus are symptom-free for a day or two after they begin spreading the virus. Once symptoms begin, adults shed virus for about five days, but children and those with impaired immune systems can do so for up to two weeks.

The most common way to catch the flu is breathing air containing the virus. Coughing or sneezing is how the virus gets into the air. Flu also can be passed when someone touches someone or something that has living virus on it. In this case, the illness usually gains access to the body from the hand by mouth, entering through the gut. Under warm and humid conditions, the influenza virus can remain infectious on surfaces like counter tops or doorknobs for a couple of days. During the winter, it can remain infectious in cold fresh water for up to a month. If you can avoid being around people sick with flu you may delay getting ill. However, if you are needed to provide care for a sick family member or friend with the virus, this strategy is not practical. Ultimately, most people are likely to be exposed to the virus. It's just a matter of time.

Wearing latex gloves and an N-95 face mask when caring for the ill and changing your clothes, mask, gloves and shoes when you leave a sick person's area is a way to protect parts of the house where healthy people live. In truth, pandemic influenza is so infectious anyone taking care of sick folks in their homes will be exposed repeatedly to the virus no matter what measures they take. Activities like helping the patient to the bathroom, changing bed linens and washing soiled clothes, or simply breathing the air in the vicinity of the sick leads to exposure. Since most people will have one or more sick family members or friends to care for during the pandemic, it is unlikely to avoid being exposes.

Coughing and hand washing etiquette

Two simple but effective suggestions for reducing spread of the virus includes covering your nose and mouth with a tissue of handkerchief when coughing or blowing your nose and washing your hands after having any contact with a sick person. Coughing or sneezing into your hands is not recommended because then you are liable to spread the virus to anything you touch with them. Instead, if a handkerchief is unavailable, cough or sneeze into the inside of your elbow or the sleeve of your upper arm. Use soap, water and a face cloth to wash your hands or you can use the new waterless alcohol gel.

The virtue of cleanliness

To help reduce the presence of virus within the home, keep sick people clean and dry. The sick rooms, bed clothing and bathrooms need to be maintained in good condition. Ventilation of these areas is important, and if possible, natural light will improve the atmosphere. Soiled garments and bedclothes need to be washed and dried, a task likely to be challenging if there is an interruption of electrical and water services. It will be important to wash these soiled items in hot water using soap and chlorine bleach if possible. Drying these items in the sun takes advantage of the powerful antiseptic effect of ultraviolet light. A good clothesline will be an essential item to have on hand.

Hard surfaces should be wiped clean using soap and water, and then sprayed with 1:10 bleach to water solution and wiped down a second time. Allow the bleach solution to stand on the surface for 30 seconds before removing it to help ensure that all the contagion is eliminated. This technique will effectively remove all trace of infectious viral particles and bacteria from surfaces that come into contact with body fluids, vomit and excrement.

Signs and Symptoms of Bird Flu

It is a bad cold or bird flu?

There are several ways to tell the difference between the flu and less severe illnesses. First of all, unless there are other cases of flu around the area, your illness is probably not flu. Colds, bronchitis, sinusitis, ear infections, and sore throat can lay you low but are less severe. Flu is a really severe illness compared with these more common conditions. So, the severity of illness is an important clue that the patient indeed has the flu. Healthy people sick with pandemic flu will be so ill and weak they will have a hard time getting up out of bed without help.

The flu usually begins in the nose with sneezing and a runny nose. A sore throat, fever and muscle aches and pains will follow. Over the next day or two, the virus will move into the lung causing cough, more fever, headache, and general weakness. If the virus gains access to the body through the gut, nausea, vomiting, abdominal cramping, and diarrhea are likely.

Principal symptoms of influenza

Fever

Everyone with flu will have a fever, which is one of the ways our bodies fight infections. Virus and bacteria don't grow as well when our body temperatures are higher than normal and our body's immune system is more active when we have a fever. So some fever is good for fighting infections. On the other hand, too much can cause damage and accelerate dehydration. The "best" temperature for balancing the benefits vs. the deficits is between 100.5° F and 101° F taken orally. If taken rectally, increase the range by ½ degree.

Cough

Almost every patient with influenza develops a cough. A wet cough is one that produces phlegm or mucus while a dry one does not. Coughing serves several useful purposes. The most important is to help clear the breathing passageways of collections of mucus or other debris that accumulate under conditions of health and disease. In this case, cough is helpful. On the other hand, when the cough is not due to mucus but instead caused by irritation on the delicate tissue lining the breathing passageways, then coughing can cause damage serving no useful purpose. The vigorous and intense contraction of the back, abdominal and rib muscles occurring repeatedly during coughing can bruise or tear them. This leads to pain when taking a breath or when these areas are pressed with the fingers. Since an excessive dry cough can be harmful, it is the one we want to suppress. On the other hand, our goal is to encourage a wet cough to help the body rid itself of mucus and debris.

In patients with infections of the ears, nose, throat, or sinuses, cough can occur when mucus from these irritated tissues finds its way down into the bronchial passageways. Cough from this cause is best treated with an antihistamine and decongestant rather than a cough suppressant. *6

The dry cough is the one we want to suppress, and the wet cough is the one we want to encourage.

Shortness of breath

When a person is short of breath, he is having a hard time getting a satisfying breath. He feels like he is not getting enough air. Sometimes this symptom is due an asthma attack or when the air passages go into a spasm of tightening. When this happens, the patient wheezes when they inhale and exhale breath. The higher the pitch of the wheeze, the more constricted the breathing tubes.

With some other causes of shortness of breath, the breathing passages are wide open, and the problem is deep in the lung being due to a buildup of fluids or pus. These are serious complications of flu. So, shortness of breath developing in a patient with flu should be evaluated by a doctor or at a hospital as soon as possible.

Pneumonia usually causes the patient to have a wet cough with lots of mucus. The mucus can be clear or colored, and can be thick or thin.

Since those who develop pneumonia during the pandemic are at high risk of dying, if at all possible, they need professional medical care.

Nausea, vomiting, and diarrhea

Vomiting and diarrhea occur when the virus affects the stomach or intestine. These flu signs cause the patient to become dehydrated quickly especially in the presence of fever. When the intestine is infected and food is eaten, it can't be digested and this leads to a worsening of the diarrhea and stomach cramps.

Signs or symptoms of serious complications of Bird Flu

Symptom or Sign	Likely Assessment	Remedy
Shortness of breath	Pneumonia	Push fluids, seek medical help
Cyanosis (skin turns blue)*7	The lung is unable to bring oxygen to the blood. This is a very bad sign and is often associated with a rapid death.	Keep the patient as comfortable as possible, seek medical help
Bleeding from mouth, coughing up blood, passing red blood per rectum. Severe bruising	A severe blood clotting disorder is present and is a very bad sign. Death is likely.	Keep the patient as comfortable as possible, seek medical help

Supportive treatment of influenza

Keeping good records

It will be useful to keep well-organized notes on the patients you are caring for at home. Having a standard approach is a good way to be sure that you have not overlooked anything of importance. Each day, write down the patient's vital signs. Include their temperature, pulse rate, breathing rate, blood pressure, and weight if they can stand. Repeat the vital signs three times daily in routine patients and more often in very sick patients. You can get a clear picture of how the patient is doing from these simple measurements. An important part of the daily record is to measure the patient's fluid intake and output. To do this, you will need to keep track of the fluid they are taking in as well as passing out. Have patients save all their urine by urinating in a chamber pot or urinal instead of the toilet. Measure the urine output using a large measuring cup. The amount of fluid we take in each day is always more than the amount passed out because of insensible losses. Insensible losses include fluid lost through the skin as perspiration, water vapor in the breath, and fluid in the stool. If the patient is not drinking enough fluid their output of urine will fall off, and the urine will become darker and concentrated. If this happens, encourage them to drink more fluids.

Identification of dehydration

When patients have a fever, vomiting, and/or diarrhea, they lose much more water from the body than is commonly appreciated. Symptoms of dehydration include weakness, dizziness, headache, confusion, and fainting. Signs of dehydration include dryness of the mouth, decreased saliva, lack of or very small urine volume that is dark and highly concentrated, sunken eyes, loss of skin elasticity, low blood pressure, especially upon sitting up or rising from the sitting to the standing position, and fast pulse rate, especially when moving from the lying to sitting or standing positions.

Preventing or treating dehydration in people with flu will save more lives than any other intervention during the influenza pandemic.

Treatment of dehydration

The Oral Rehydration Solution (ORS) is an excellent treatment for all causes of dehydration. It is just what the thirsty body needs to restore the lost fluid. The water, salt and sugar in the formula team up to speed the patient's recovery. The quantity of sugar in the ORS can be varied depending on the patient preference. It can be increased up to 4 tbsp or reduced to 2 tbsp if desired by the patient. For some people, the ORS will taste too salty. In this case, increase the water content to 1.5 or even 2 quarts leaving the remainder of the formula unchanged.

The Adult ORS formula for dehydration
    1 quart clean water
    1 level tsp table salt
    3 tbsp table sugar

If you detect or suspect that dehydration is developing, administer the ORS by mouth. If the patient is too ill to drink, someone must sit with them and administer the fluids using a teaspoon or a baby bottle to get one spoonful or dribble from the bottle down the patient's throat until she is strong enough to drink alone. Don't stop until the patient has been able to keep down at least a quart of fluids, which my take several hours. You will know you are making headway with fluid therapy when the patient becomes more alert and begins urinating, an indication that their fluid deficit is partially restored. While these are good signs, more remains to be done. With sick patients like these, you need to "push the fluids" so don't let your guard down. If they are too weak to use a glass and straw or squeeze bottle, try an 8oz. baby bottle, which may be easier to handle. Your patient will be very tired. Let them sleep for a couple of hours and then get them to drink more fluids. Be insistent, it is really important.

You can drink the ORS plain or add fruit flavorings or natural herbs like tea, vanilla, cloves, cinnamon or mint. A number of excellent powdered fruit drink products are available at the grocery store that can be mixed with the ORS. Once the patient is well hydrated and eating, there is no further need for the ORS. Even if the patient is not eating but can drink and remains well hydrated, you can switch them to one of the other fluids listed for use with the clear liquid diet such as juice, bouillon or tea.

Treatment of common flu symptoms
Caring for a flu patient is something everyone is capable of doing. The basic goals are to keep the patient clean, dry, warm and well hydrated. Patients need a soft place to lie down, be comforted, told that they are going to be OK, and reassured that you will be there for them. The most important medical treatment is to make sure they have plenty of fluids. Dehydration must be prevented because it can quickly lead to death or contribute to stroke or heart attack. Keeping the patient hydrated is the best treatment for the flu and the one that is most likely to save lives. The

same treatment advice applies to other viral and bacterial illnesses that might be confused with influenza. So, don't worry so much about whether or not you have made the correct diagnosis or not. The treatment will be about the same anyway.

Treatment of adults with fever

The first consideration when treating a patient with fever is fluid therapy. It is very difficult to bring a fever down in a patient low on fluids. Both ibuprofen and acetaminophen are good ways to lower fever and help the patient feel better. The therapeutic dose of ibuprofen for adults is 2 to 4 tablets (400mg to 800mg) every four to six hours as needed. *8 For acetaminophen, the dose is two 500mg tablets up to four times daily as needed. Try one or the other at the dose recommended. Wait 45 minutes. If the response is insufficient, add a full dose of the other drug. In adults, acetaminophen and ibuprofen can be used in full doses at the same time, because they are in different drug classes and have different drug side effects. Combination treatment with both has an additive effect of benefit without increasing risk. Do not exceed these doses for either drug. This is the maximum for both. Acetaminophen is a very safe drug as long as you do not exceed the daily dose limit for it.

Many cold and flu preparations sold in drug stores include acetaminophen or ibuprofen along with antihistamines and or decongestants. These are fine to use for flu. Just remember to include the dose of acetaminophen and ibuprofen found in these drugs in your daily limit calculation to avoid exceeding it for any of the drugs listed.

A high fever (103° F) is hard on the patient, but most folks can tolerate it well. A fever above 104° F is the upper safe limit for most people and anything above 105° F is a temperature emergency. Fevers this high can cause seizures and above this point brain damage can develop if prolonged. This must be avoided. The mainstays of therapy are keeping the patient well-hydrated, tepid water sponge baths, acetaminophen, ibuprofen and dressing the patient lightly.

If the fever resists these techniques, sponge bathe the patient with cool water and fan the patient to increase the cooling effect of evaporation from the skin. As a last resort, if you have access to either ice or snow, make cold packs and place them under each arm, on the right and left sides of the groin, around the neck. These cold packs cool the blood passing under them helping to reduce the patient's temperature.

Treatment of chills and body aches and pains
Chills cause shivering and are often associated with body aches and later fever. Treat chills by keeping the patient warm; give them an extra blanket or a hot water bottle. Body aches respond to acetaminophen, and ibuprofen used separately or together.

Treatment for respiratory conditions and headache
Gargling with a hot salt and soda water solution is a good treatment for sore throat. To make this treatment, add 1 tsp of salt and ¼ tsp of baking soda to a cup of hot but not scalding water. Ibuprofen and acetaminophen used in full doses either individually or together if needed have good pain relieving effects.

Nasal, sinus and ear congestion and pain respond to hot packs placed on the face and by inhaling steamy air. Use of a salt and soda saline solution to wash the sinuses helps remove mucus and inflammatory chemicals that build up in the area and is very useful. The solution is made by adding ¼ level tsp of table salt plus ¼ level tsp of baking soda to 1 cup of clean water. Instill the solution into the nose with an ear bulb syringe or by other means and gently blow your nose. Repeat this process until the nasal passage is clear. Nasal washing can be repeated as often as needed. Antihistamines and decongestants are also useful for treatment of this condition. The salt and soda saline solution makes an excellent non-burning eye wash too. It is a great way to provide a comforting bath to sore runny eyes and lids.

Inhaling steamy air is a time-honored therapy for chest, sinus, ear and throat infections. The easiest way to create steam is by heating water in a teakettle or a pot. Once the water is boiling, drape a towel over your head and bend over near but not too close to the steam. Inhale the steamy air through the nose and mouth getting it deep into the lungs.

From the therapeutic standpoint, we want to encourage patients with a wet cough to clear the mucus from their lungs. The health of the patient is unaffected if the phlegm brought up with a wet cough is swallowed or deposited in a handkerchief. Hydrating the patient with the ORS, feeding them a hot or cold caffeine-containing beverage like tea, coffee, or cola, or eating chocolate encourages a wet cough.

Reasons and remedies for common flu patient signs and symptoms I

Symptoms or Sign	Likely Assessment	Remedy
Low urine output	Dehydration	Give the patient ORS
High pulse rate >90	Dehydration or fever	Give the patient ORS
Shaking chills and shivers	The virus is swarming in the blood stream	Keep the patient warm
Nausea/Vomiting	The virus is affecting stomach or indirectly the brain	Give sips of clear liquid diet. Use the ORS. Use meclizine 25mg every 4 hours as needed
Diarrhea	The virus is affecting intestine	Push ORS fluids, clear liquid diet
Severe stomach cramps	The virus is affecting the intestine. Expect nausea, vomiting and diarrhea soon	Switch to clear liquid diet. Use diphenhydramine and/or loperamide for cramps
Bloody diarrhea but no bleeding from any other site	The virus has infected the intestinal lining	Push ORS fluids and use the clear liquid diet. Give loperamide and/or diphenhydramine for cramps

The cough reflex is effectively suppressed with dextromethorphan, the drug found in many OTC cough products with the "DM" notation on their label. If the patient has a wet cough and is coughing a lot, you still should suppress it to prevent the cough from damaging the chest wall or lung structures. Too much coughing, even when bringing up phlegm, can cause damage and should be lessened. Inhaling warm humidified air helps patients with infections of the nose, sinus, ears, throat, bronchial pathways, and lungs especially during winter when the air is dry. Caffeinated tea and coffee and chocolate contain an herb with well known medicinal effects on the lungs. The herb helps keep the breathing tubes open, increase heart rate and blood flow, and encourage urination. The effect is to move more fluid through the lungs thinning the mucus and making it easier to cough up. The herb is also effective for relieving headache, lifting a depressed mood and for enhancing awareness.

Chest pain during flu is often due to the effect of coughing on the muscles, ribs and cartilages that surround and support the lungs. An indication of this cause is when pressing on the chest wall, upper flanks, or upper abdomen brings out the pain. Treatment is to suppress the cough as explained above, allowing these injured tissues to heal. Pain can be controlled using a full dose acetaminophen and/or ibuprofen every six hours. Muscle spasm can play a role in this pain, and when it does, consider applying an icepack, heating pad, or hot water bottle to the chest wall. Chest pain can be excruciatingly painful and difficult to control.

Reasons and remedies for common flu patient signs and symptoms II

Symptom or Sign	Likely Assessment	Remedy
Headache	Due to fever or coughing. Also can be directly or indirectly due to the viral infection	Ibuprofen and/or acetaminophen. Lower temperature if fever present. Use icepack on neck.
Fever	Due to the virus stimulating the bodies immune system to release chemicals that fight the infection	Ibuprofen, acetaminophen, push fluids, keep warm or cool, consider tepid water baths if > 102° F OK if < 101° F as this may help kill virus
Sore throat	Direct viral infection of the posterior throat tissue. Caused by inflammation of tissue breakdown in the area	Gargle with hot salt water, drink hot tea or hot water, ibuprofen and or acetaminophen
Cough	Viral infection and irritation of the tissue lining the breathing tubes	Push the ORS fluids, drink hot tea for effect on breathing tubes, use a

	and/or the lung tissue	dextromethorphan (DM) containing cough syrup to suppress cough if needed
Facial pain	Sinus congestion or infection	Use salt and soda nasal solution frequently, hot packs or cold packs on face help, diphenhydramine 25-50mg four times daily as an antihistamine and ibuprofen and/or Tylenol for pain. Push fluids including tea
Runny nose	Virus infecting nose	Use salt and soda nasal solution frequently, diphenhydramine 25-50mg four times daily to reduce runny nose

Headache with influenza can come from several sources. Coughing shakes the head back and forth and can strain the neck muscles causing headache. Chemicals released by the viral infected cells and the immune system can trigger headaches. Bacterial sinusitis complicating flu causes facial pain and headache. Treat headaches using ibuprofen with or without acetaminophen. If neck stiffness or soreness is present, apply an ice pack, heating pad, or hot water bottle to the back of the neck or head.

Treatment of nausea, vomiting, diarrhea and abdominal pain

The first step in treatment for these four symptoms is to place the patient on a clear liquid diet using the ORS. It will not provoke vomiting or diarrhea as easily as other fluids or foods do, but it can still cause these reactions in severely affected people. Nausea is responsive to meclizine 25-50mg every 4 to 6 hours as needed for this symptom. Diarrhea and abdominal cramping can be treated with diphenhydramine 25-50mg every 4 to 6 hours and/or loperamide 2 – 4 mg every 4 to 6 hours. Since diphenhydramine and meclizine are both antihistamines, their side effects are additive. If you have already given the patient one of these drugs and want to try the other, wait four hours before doing so to allow the first drug to clear the system.

Patients with an intestinal presentation of flu often will experience abdominal cramping, gas, and diarrhea. In some patients, the diarrhea can be bloody. Diarrhea often causes irritation around the anus. Treat this by gently cleaning the area using a moistened tissue, soft cloth or baby wipe. Apply a small amount of petroleum jelly or cocoa butter on and around the anus to protect and heal the tissue. Repeat this process after each loose stool. Abdominal cramps response to the anticholinergic effects of diphenhydramine 12.5 to 25mg every four to six hours.

Diet and Exercise with Influenza

Since flu commonly takes away the appetite, most patients won't be hungry. Eating is not as important as drinking fluids because the patient will be breaking down muscle and fat for energy. The clear liquid diet is best for patients sick with flu who are not particularly hungry, but it is mandatory for patients with diarrhea due to influenza. If a flu patient wants to eat, feed them as long as they don't have diarrhea. In most cases, patients with diarrhea can tolerate a clear liquid diet without making matters worse. The small intestine can absorb water, minerals, and sugars well even when infected.

If the patient has not been sick long or had a mild non-diarrheal presentation of the flu, you can start with step 2 of the clear liquid diet and quickly move up the steps as tolerated by the patient. At any time during re-feeding, should the patient suffer abdominal problems, especially pain or diarrhea, drop back a step or two on the clear liquid diet. Rest in that step for a while before trying the next step again. This strategy will work well for almost every patient.

The clear liquid diet

1. Oral Rehydration Solution (ORS), water, fruit juice, Jell-O, Gatorade, Popsicles, PowerAde, ginger ale, cola, tea, and bouillon.
2. To Step 1 add white toast (no butter or oils), white rice, cream of wheat, soda crackers, and potatoes without the skin.
3. To Step 2 add canned fruit and chicken noodle soup.
4. To Step 3 add a source of protein like canned meat, fish or egg.

5. To Step 4 add milk and other dairy products, vegetable oils, butter, raw fruits and vegetables and high fiber whole grain products.

Once the patient is eating a normal diet without any stomach problems, it is important to increase the intake of high quality protein, especially eggs, meat, fish, or poultry. This nutrition is needed to rebuild the muscle and organ tissues, which were broken down for energy during the illness. Carbohydrates and fats are also important as an energy source for the recovering body and to help replace lost fat stores broken down for energy during the infection.

Exercise during and after recovery

Even moderate influenza causes a breakdown of muscle tissue and physical weakness. If a patient was critically ill with the flu, even more muscle, organ tissue, and fat was broken down by the body for support. Acute influenza symptoms can be expected to last at least five days but usually seven to 10 days. Most people need another week or two of rest for recovery. A return to limited normal activities is usually possible at this time, but full recovery will not be complete for a month or even two, after the infection. Of course, no exercise of any type is possible or desirable during the acute phase of the illness. During the recovery period, passive stretching and massage helps a weakened patient recover. These activities help bring the dormant joints, tendons, and muscles back to life and work out the soreness that builds up in these tissues. Gentle passive range of motion (ROM) exercise is accomplished by slowly and repeatedly moving all the joints of the limbs, including fingers and toes, through their entire normal range of movement. Each finger and toe, ankles, knees, hips, wrists, elbows, shoulders, and the neck should be bent, rotated, and extended slowly and repeatedly. Gentle massage is also comforting to the patient's sore muscles and helps in their recovery.

Patients who have been at bed rest for a long time will have trouble with balance and weakness. If they have not been eating, they will not have enough energy to resume normal activity. A prerequisite for getting up is to get the patient past step 3 of the clear liquid diet before even trying to encourage the patient to walk again.

When the time comes to help a patient return to normal, take it easy. Try sitting the patient upright in bed first. If this goes well, the patient can next try sitting on the side of the bed with his feet on the floor. Dizziness and weakness are the two problems that most people have trouble overcoming. Take it slowly. Dizziness usually goes away after a while in this position, so be patient. The next step is to get the patient up and sitting in a chair. Standing with limited assisted walking comes next. At first, have the patient walk with assistance around the room or in the halls.

Home Care of Children with Flu

Many differences exist between the way a child and an adult respond to this disease. Many, but not all, of the drugs used for adults are also used for children, but the dose is different. Dehydration and rehydration are critical in both, except that children can become dehydrated much more quickly than adults. While many of the recommendations and advice for treatment of adults can be applied to kids, some are inappropriate. A wise parent will ask their children's pediatrician for flu management suggestions for use during the pandemic before it begins. Your pediatrician knows your child's health better than anyone, and the advice and counsel of your doctor take precedence over any suggestions presented here.

Signs and symptoms of flu in children

One of the biggest challenges for patents will be trying to tell whether their sick child has a cold or bird flu. If bird flu is not in your community, it is very unlikely that your child will be the first case. It is common for the first signs of flu to be a runny nose followed by irritability or crankiness. A sore throat and fever often follow. When the virus moves down into the lung, dry cough begins. Infants with influenza can suddenly become very sick rapidly or simply "not look right". They may seem unresponsive, dull eyed, and distant. One difference between a cold and flu is in the speed with which the flu strikes a child compared with a slow-moving cold. Also, flu is much more severe than a cold. If the child is running around as usual and eating normally, he probably doesn't have flu or is in the very early stages of the illness.

These symptoms are not specific for flu so when they develop, keep calm and treat them in the same way you would manage any cold—with fluids, acetaminophen and rest. If flu is in your community and the disease course is more or less following the above pattern, flu becomes more likely but is still unproven. The feature that makes flu so different from routine childhood infectious diseases is the severity of the illness. Kids with pandemic bird flu will be very sick very fast. Its quick onset and the severity of the illness are what clearly distinguished flu from a cold.

Signs and symptoms of influenza in children

Fever	Sore throat	Loss of appetite
Cough	Runny nose	Headache
Dizziness	Weakness	Irritability
Muscles aches	Nausea	Vomiting
Chills	Ear pain	Fatigue
Diarrhea	Crying for no reason	

How to keep children with flu comfortable

- A child with flu should gets lots of rest, which will help her body fight the virus, and keep her more comfortable.
- Use the ORS to provide her with plenty of fluids. Being well hydrated is the easiest way to make nasal mucous thinner, relieve stuffy noses, and soothe sore throats.
- Use a cool mist humidifier in your child's bedroom to reduce coughing, which often gets worse at night.
- Use a nasal aspirator (a syringe that sucks mucus from the nostrils) or ear bulb syringe along with the salt and soda nose spray to relieve stuffy noses in smaller children and infants.
- Older toddlers can be taught to blow their noses.
- For smaller children, raise the head of the crib (with a book or pillow under the mattress) to ease congestion and coughing.
- Use acetaminophen for fever, aches, or pains.
- Use a DM (Dextromethorphan) containing cough syrup for cough. *9

Dehydration in Children

Dehydration presents in children in the same manner as in adults, only more quickly because children have less body water. This means they can become dangerously low on fluids very quickly especially if diarrhea or vomiting accompanies the fever.

Signs and symptoms of dehydration in children

Early in dehydration, a child may be cranky and irritable. Later lethargy or lifelessness may develop. A lethargic child is difficult to awaken. They have very little energy and are "rag doll weak". Sunken eyes, dry nose or mouth and decreased or absent urination are very worrisome signs that indicate the development of dehydration. The heart rate is fast when the child is feverish, but it is also fast when the child is dehydrated. A dehydrated child may have a glassy-eyed stare and have difficulty focusing or concentrating. This is never normal and should be considered a sign the child is very ill and probably needs fluids. Failure to effectively treat dehydration will make it nearly impossible to bring a fever down to a safe level. If dehydration continues unchecked, eventually the child will go into shock and die.

Signs and symptoms of dehydration in children

Sunken eyes	Decreased urination or dry diapers
Sunken skull "soft spot" fontanel in infants	Tearless crying
Dry mouth or sticky mucus membranes	Lethargy, reduced movement, fussiness
Irritability buy may be "too tired to cry"	

Treatment of flu symptoms in children

Prevention of dehydration

Since several common flu symptoms and signs cause dehydration, you should assume that it will develop unless you take steps to prevent it. This is the best strategy. As soon as the child becomes ill, begin fluid therapy and keep pushing the fluids as long as she has a fever, diarrhea, or is not eating.

Correction of dehydration in children

Fluid treatment is indicated for dehydration whether from flu or another cause. If nothing comes of the symptoms, fluid therapy is harmless. The principles of rehydration used in adults are the same as for children but the ORS formula is a little different. Be persistent in your efforts to get as much fluid in the child as you can.

Children's ORS Formula for dehydration

1.5 quarts clean water
1 level tsp. table salt
4 tbsp. table sugar

Treatment of cough

Almost every child with bird flu will cough. Cough has a useful purpose, to help rid the lung of mucus and phlegm. A dry cough is usually due to an irritated breathing passage. In this case, cough makes things worse not better. IF persistent, the coughing can bruise the voice box and breathing tubes in the lung. These bruises cause pain when breathing. In the case of a dry cough due to flu, use of a cough syrup containing dextromethorphan (DM) is helpful. This drug can cause hallucinations if given for more than several days or in high doses. Keeping the child hydrated is very important for treatment of cough. Another useful technique is humidified air. Using a room humidifier is useful if available.

If mucus comes up with the cough, this is known as a wet cough. We want to encourage a wet cough to help the child clear the mucus from the lung but too much coughing can damage the lung and chest and stomach muscles. So in some cases, use of a little cough suppressing cough syrup is useful for an aggressive wet cough.

Treatment of runny nose

The best treatment for runny nose is use of salt and soda saline solution made of 1/4 tsp. of salt and ¼ tsp. of baking soda added to a cup of clean water. The best approach is to spray the solution into the nose as a mist. Alternatively, an ear bulb syringe works well for this purpose. The salt and soda solution will help remove mucus and irritants that clog the nasal passage and will help these tissues heal. Use of good nose blowing technique by the child is important to successful nasal solution use. Teach children to wash their hands after they blow their nose or cough into a handkerchief.

Antihistamines are an effective treatment for runny nose. Diphenhydramine, the generic name for Benadryl, is an antihistamine recognized as safe and effective in children. Commercial children's Benadryl is widely available as an oral tablet that melts in the child's mouth. This product is easy to use and a good treatment for runny nose. Oral diphenhydramine has few side effects including its tendency to sedate. This side effect actually can be an advantage if the child needs help in sleeping. Sometimes people have an atypical hyperactive response to antihistamines, and if this is the case, they should be avoided, especially in children.

Treatment of fever in children

Children can mount impressive fevers quite suddenly. It is common for fever to go up and down during the day and night. Aches and pains parallel the fever. Fevers can have a daily pattern, and it is common for a child's temperature to reach 104° F during a severe infection. A goal of therapy is to lower the fever to between 100.5° F and 101° F, where the body's immune system is most effective at eliminating the infection. If the temperature rises above 105° F, seizures or even brain injury are possible. So, it is important to aggressively manage the child's fever before it becomes extreme.

Restoring fluid losses due to fever or other causes is always the first step in treatment of fever. Failure to restore the child's fluid volume will make it nearly impossible to lower the temperature. Acetaminophen reduces temperature and helps with aches and pains. Be sure to use it in full children's doses rather than partial doses. Use the weight and age-based dose guidelines provided with the children's acetaminophen product. A tepid water sponge bath is a useful method in lowering fever. Never give a child or an adult an alcohol sponge bath, which can be toxic. In rare instances, using all the methods above fails to lower the temperature to below 101 F. In this case, lower the temperature of the water you use for the sponge bath or fan the child to speed the evaporation of fluid from the body. An additional measure, if absolutely necessary, is to place ice or snow packs in plastic zip lock-type bags wrapped in kitchen towels under both arms, around the neck, and between the legs on the groin. High volumes of blood are cooled with this technique as it passes by these areas. This method is difficult for the child, but it is a fast way to lower core body temperature in an emergency.

How to take your child's temperature accurately *12

To measure your child's fever accurately use:

- A rectal or tympanic (ear) thermometer for children less than 3 years old
- A digital (not glass) oral thermometer for children over 3 years
- Avoid using an ear thermometer until your baby is at least 3 months old. It may not be accurate, because young infants have such narrow ear canals.

Temperature readings are different from different parts of the body (rectum, ear, mouth). Your child has a fever if her temperature is above:

- Rectal 100.4° F
- Oral 99.5° F
- Axillary (underarm) 98.6° F
- Tympanic (ear) 100.0° F

Keeping your child comfortable with a fever

- If the child is shivering, keep her warm until the shivering stops
- If the child is not shivering, you can remove her warm clothes and encourage her to drink plenty of fluids.
- Keep your child rested, quiet, and comfortable in a cool room.
- Place a cool washcloth on your child's forehead or sponge her with tepid water. Stop if you child starts to shiver.
- Never use rubbing alcohol to cool your child's skin – the vapors are toxic and can be absorbed through the skin.
- Acetaminophen in children's doses is a safe and effective way to lower the fever in kids. It takes from 30 to 60 minutes to begin working.
- Monitor your child's temperature, appearance, and behavior periodically – keeping an eye out for signs of a more serious illness – until she seems to be back to normal.

Treatment of nausea, vomiting and diarrhea in children

The most important treatment for nausea, vomiting, cramping and diarrhea is to stop feeding the child and place them on a clear liquid diet. Start with Oral Rehydration Solution plain or with a little powdered fruit-flavored drink mix for taste. Give the child small amounts of the ORS solution in sips from the baby bottle. This will help prevent dehydration and is not likely to make cramping worse. Meclizine 25mg given every 4 to 6 hours can help reduce nausea in children age 12 years and older. It is not US FDA approved for use in younger children.

To stop diarrhea, consider using a small dose of the diphenhydramine. The anticholinergic effect of this drug will calm the intestine. Use a low, age/weight appropriate dose every four to six hours as needed. For children over age 2 years, loperamide 1 to2 mg every 4 to 6 hours can be used for diarrhea and abdominal cramping.

Acetaminophen use in children

Acetaminophen, best known as the brand name product Tylenol, is an excellent drug for treatment of pain and fever in children from toddlers to teens. It also helps children sleep when given at bedtime. It is very safe with the only issue related to total daily dose, which must not be exceeded to prevent liver injury. In children, the safe dose limit changes with age and weight. The younger a child or the smaller, the lower the safe dose limits. The easiest thing to do is use Johnson and Johnson's brand name Children's Tylenol or Infant's Concentrated Drops or the identical generic drugstore brand of these products.

References
1. The patients will find it much easier to drink fluids from a baby bottle, squeeze bottle, or using a straw during their illness.
2. Use a teakettle for making tea and as a device for making steam for treatment of sinus and bronchial disorders.
3. Petroleum jelly will be useful for chapped lips, noses and bottoms
4. Use cocoa butter to make rectal or vaginal suppositories. It is also an outstanding lip balm and great treatment for chapped or irritated skin of the nose or perianal area.
5. Thermometers break so have more than one on hand.

6. Fever, cough and shortness of breath are the three most common symptoms of Bird Flu in patients' admitted to the hospital with the disease in Southeast Asia from 2003 through July 2005. Adapted from: Avian Influenza A (H5N1) Infection in Humans. N. Engl. J Med 2005: 353:1374-1385

7. During the 1918 pandemic a particularly aggressive presentation of influenza that was most commonly seen in young adults was associated with cyanosis and is described in this excerpt from a physician's letter to a colleague. "After a few hours later you can begin to see the Cyanosis extending from their ears and spreading all over the face, until it is hard to distinguish the colored men from the white. It is only a matter of a few hours then until death comes."

8. For the purposed of this book, ibuprofen means aspirin, Advin, Aleve, ibuprofen, or Nuprin since they are all alike. Acetaminophen (Tylenol) is not an aspirin.

9. Dextromethorphan HBr is an antitussive (cough suppressant) that inhibits the cough reflex. It acts primarily by depressing the cough center in the brain to reduce the frequency of the intensity of cough. Prolonged use or high doses can cause confusion or hallucinations. DM is not a very strong cough suppressant.

10. Adapted from a chart found on Johnson and Johnson's Tylenol web site.

About the Author

Grattan Woodson, MD practices internal medicine at the Druid Oaks Health Center in Decatur, GA. He became concerned about avian influenza after learning about the first human cases in Hong Kong in 1997. His interest grew when the disease re-emerged in 2003-04 and he began to study in earnest. His work led to the conclusion that humankind was about to be visited again by a severe influenza pandemic resembling the 1918 Spanish Influenza. In order to help prepare his patients for this possibility, he began writing on this topic, which ultimately resulted in the publication of two books, *The Bird Flue Preparedness Planner* in November 2005 and *The Bird Flu Manual* in September 2006.

Section II

Recipes

Clear Liquid Diet

Step 1: Oral Rehydration Solution, water fruit juice, Jell-O, Gatorade, Popsicles, PowerAde, ginger ale, cola, tea and bouillon.

Step 2: To Step 1 add white toast (no butter or oils), white rice, cream of wheat, soda crackers, and potatoes without the skin.

Step 3: To Step 2 add canned fruit and chicken noodle soup.

Step 4: To Step 3 add a source of protein like canned meat, fish or egg.

Step 5: To Step 4 add milk and other dairy products, vegetable oils, butter, raw fruit and vegetables and high fiber whole grain products.

Electrolyte Replacer

½ tsp. Table Salt
¼ tsp. Salt Substitute (or Potassium Chloride)
½ tsp. Baking Soda
2 tbsp. Sugar

Mix everything together with 1 quart boiling water. Cool to serve.

You may add 1 package unsweetened kool-aid or 1 packet of Emergen-C to mixture for flavor and added vitamins (Emergen-C).

Emergency Baby Formula

Evaporated Milk Version

2 C. boiled water (cooled)
1 Can (13 oz.) evaporated milk
2 Tbsp. Karo Syrup

Stir until well blended. Pour into a sterilized jar or bottle and store in the refrigerator until needed.

Powdered Milk Version

2 2/3 C. prepared powdered milk (made with boiled water)
2 Tbsp. Karo Syrup

Stir until well blended. Pour into a sterilized jar or bottle and store in the refrigerator until needed.

Lice Shampoo

Natural Lice Shampoo

5 tsp. Pure Olive Oil (or Pure Coconut Oil)
5 drops Tea Tree Essential Oil
5 drops Rosemary Essential Oil
5 drops Lavender Essential Oil
5 drops Peppermint Essential Oil
5 drops Eucalyptus Essential Oil

Add a small amount of regular shampoo to the mixture and massage through hair. Leave on hair for an hour under a towel or tight-fitting shower cap to prevent drips. Rinse the hair and shampoo the hair.

(The olive oil or coconut oil kill lice by dissolving their exoskeletons – other oils will not have the same effect)

NOTE: 1) The respiration of a baby or child under 5 can be slowed down or even stopped if peppermint oil or eucalyptus oil is close enough for the baby to breathe. 2) High blood pressure may be elevated by peppermint essential oil. 3) Peppermint or rosemary may be harmful during pregnancy. In any of these cases, just use the recipe without the oil that may be harmful in your case.

Oral Rehydration Therapy

ORT 1
1 Liter (quart) boiled water
1 teaspoon salt
8 teaspoons sugar
1 mashed banana (for potassium and improved taste) Optional

If you leave out banana, replace with potassium chloride.

CAUTION: Before adding the sugar, taste the drink and be sure it is less salty than tears.

ORT 2
1 Liter (quart) boiled water
½ teaspoon salt
8 heaping teaspoons of cereal (finely ground maize, wheat flour, sorghum or cooked and mashed potatoes

Boil for 5 to 7 minutes to form a liquid gruel or watery porridge. Cool the drink quickly and start administering.

CAUTION: Taste the drink each time it is used to be sure it is not spoiled. Cereal drinks can spoil in a few hours in hot weather.

*To either drink add Potassium Chloride or half a cup of fruit juice, coconut water or mashed ripe banana, if available. This provides potassium, which may help the person accept more food and drink.

Starvation Fluids

Starvation Fluids

½ C dried skim milk (prepared with water)
1/3 C edible oil
¼ C Sugar

Mix together adding ground up vitamins if available. Feed frequently throughout the first 24 hours of treatment.

Saline Solution

Fill a clean quart jar with freshly boiled water

Add 2 - 3 heaping teaspoons pickling/canning salt (not iodized)

Add 1 teaspoon baking soda

Stir or shake before each use

Discard after 1 week

Section III

Treatment of Symptoms

Cough

Description
What is it?

A cough can be categorized into two types, dry (non-productive) and chesty (productive). A dry cough occurs when the throat and upper airway become inflamed and swollen. A cough that doesn't produce any mucus or phlegm is a dry cough. A chesty cough is a mucus producing cough. Most coughs are acute in nature. They appear suddenly and most often do not last more than 2 to 3 weeks.

Treatment
How do I care for my patient?

Humidity
- Drape a towel over your head and inhale the steam from a bowl of steaming hot water three to four times a day. The steam will sooth the swollen and irritated throat and airway.

Liquids
- Hot drinks and soups soothe the throat. Chicken soup not only soothes, but has antiviral properties. Hot water with lemon and honey added soothes and coats the throat.

Gargle
- Gargles are always effective for easing a dry cough. Add some salt to a glass of warm water and gargle.

Caution

When the patient has a chesty cough, they should be encouraged to expel the mucus or phlegm rather than suppress the cough.

Dehydration/Diarrhea

Description
What is it?

Dehydration results when the body loses more liquid than it takes in. This can happen with severe diarrhea, especially when there is vomiting too. It can happen in very serious illness or when a person is too sick to take much food or liquid. Anyone can become dehydrated **but it develops more quickly and is most dangerous in small children.**

Treatment
How do I care for my patient?

When a person has watery diarrhea, or diarrhea and vomiting, do not wait for signs of dehydration – **Act quickly:**

- Give lots of liquids to drink: Rehydration Drink is best; or give a thin cereal porridge or gruel, teas, soups, or even plain water.
- Keep giving food: As soon as the person will accept food, give frequent feeding of foods he likes – will accept.
- For babies – keep giving breast milk often – and before other drinks.

Give the dehydrated person sips of this Drink every 5 minutes, day and night, until he begins to urinate normally. A large person needs 3 or more liters a day. A small child usually needs at least 1 liter a day, or 1 glass for each watery stool. Keep giving the Drink often in small sips, even if the person vomits. Not all of the Drink will be vomited.

Earache

Description
What is it?

An earache usually accompanies a bad cold or sore throat. The reason this happens is because fluids build up in the Eustachian tubes. The fluid becomes infected and builds up in the back of the eardrum and puts pressure on the ear.

Treatment
How do I care for my patient?
Garlic

- Puncture a piece of garlic, squeeze the juice out of it and pour the juice in the ear that hurts. Garlic is a known natural antibiotic. Stop using if a skin rash occurs.

Oils

- Slightly warm a few drops of olive or mineral oil and pour into the sore ear. The oil will act as a lubricant and may help to eliminate the dry, itchy symptoms of an ear infection. Apply the warm oil with an ear or eye dropper. Use only enough oil to coat the inner lining of the ear.
- Blend a clove of garlic with 3 tablespoons of olive oil until they are liquid, heat and pour into affected ear.
- Warmed mullein oil dropped into the ear canal is comforting.

Hot water bottle

- Wrap a hot water bottle in a towel. Use the wrapped hot water bottle as a pillow by laying the sore ear on it.

Sit up

- When suffering from an earache, you are better off sitting up instead of laying down.

Caution

If you see any blood or pus in your ear or have dizzy spells or swelling, do not put any oils or foreign substances in your ear. You may very well have burst an ear drum. In that case, the pain should subside quickly and healing will begin.

Fever

Description
What is it?

When a person's body temperature is too hot, he has a fever. Fever is not a sickness, but a sign of many different sicknesses.

Signs/Symptoms
What does it look like?

A high fever (over 39° C or over 102° F) can be dangerous, especially in a small child.

Treatment
How do I care for my patient?

When a person has a fever:

1. Uncover him completely. Small children should be undressed completely and let naked until the fever goes down. **Never** wrap the child in clothing or blankets. **To wrap up a child with fever is dangerous.** Fresh air or a breeze will not harm a person with fever. On the contrary, a fresh breeze helps lower the fever.
2. Take aspirin to lower fever. For small children, it is safer to give acetaminophen (Tylenol). Be careful not to give too much.
3. Anyone who has a fever should drink lots of water, juices, or other liquids. For small children, especially babies, drinking water should be boiled first (and then cooled). Make sure the child passes urine regularly. If she does not pass much urine, or the urine is dark, give a lot more water.
4. When possible, find and treat the cause of the fever.

Very high fevers

A very high fever can be dangerous if it is not brought down soon. It can cause seizures (convulsions) or even permanent brain damage (paralysis, mental slowness, epilepsy, etc.). High fever is most dangerous for small children.

When a fever goes very high **(over 40° C or over 104° F)**, it must be lowered at once:
1. Put the person in a cool place.
2. Remove all clothing.
3. Fan him/her.
4. Pour cool (not cold) water over him, or put cloths soaked in cool water on his chest and forehead. Fan the cloths and change the often to keep them cool. Continue to do this until the fever goes down (below 101° F).
5. Give him plenty of cool (not cold) water to drink.
6. Give a medicine to bring down fever. Aspirin or acetaminophen (Tylenol) works well.

Dosage for acetaminophen (Tylenol) or aspirin (using 300 mg. adult tablets):
- Persons over 12 years: 2 tablets every 4 hours
- Children 6 to 12 years: 1 tablet every 4 hours
- Children 3 to 6 years: ½ tablet every 4 hours
- Children under 3 years: ¼ tablet every 4 hours

Note: Acetaminophen (Tylenol) is safer than aspirin for a child under 12 years old who has a cold, flu, or chickenpox.

If a person with fever cannot swallow the tablets, grind them up, mix the powder with some water, and put it up the anus as an enema or with a syringe without the needle.

Shock

Description
What is it?

Shock is a life threatening condition that can result from a large burn, losing a lot of blood, severe illnesses, dehydration, or severe allergic reaction. Heavy bleeding inside the body – although not seen – can also cause shock.

Signs/Symptoms
What does it look like?

- Weak, rapid pulse (more than 100 beats per minute)
- 'cold sweat'; pale, cold, damp skin
- Blood pressure drops dangerously low
- Mental confusion, weakness, or loss of consciousness

Treatment/Prevention
How do I care for my patient?

At the first sign of shock, or if there is risk of shock.......

- Loosen any belts or tight clothing the person may be wearing.
- Have the person lie down with his feet a little higher than his head. (Can put blocks under the legs of the foot of the bed or cot) However, if he has a severe head injury, put him/her in a "half sitting position". (Place pillows behind person's back)
- Stop any bleeding. Use gloves or a plastic bag to keep the blood off your hands.
- If the person feels cold, cover him with a blanket.
- If he is conscious and able to drink, give him sips of water or other drinks. If he looks dehydrated, give a lot of liquid, and Rehydration Drink. If he does not respond quickly, give intravenous fluids if you know how.

- Treat his wounds, if he has any. If he is in pain, give him aspirin or another pain medicine – but **not** one with a sedative such as codeine.
- Keep calm, reassure the person, and seek medical help.

If the person is unconscious:

- Lay him on his side with his head low. If he seems to be choking, pull his tongue forward with your finger.
- If he has vomited, clear his mouth immediately. Be sure his head is low, tilted back, and to one side so he does not breathe vomit into his lungs. If he has a neck or spine injury, do not tilt his head or move his back.
- Do not give him anything by mouth until he becomes conscious.
- If you or someone nearby knows how, give intravenous solution (normal saline) at a fast drip.
- Seek medical help fast.

Sore Throat

Description
What is it?

A sore throat accompanies any number of ailments. Often, it is associated with the common cold, due to breathing with your mouth open or post-nasal drip. Occasionally, it is the symptom of a more serious illness, such as Strep throat.

Treatment
How do I care for my patient?

Most sore throats are easily treatable with simple home remedies, the most common of which are;

Gargle
- Gargling with warm water (8oz.) and salt (1 tsp.) offer quick relief. Gargle often for pain.
- Gargling with Apple Cider Vinegar (ACV) is a known to quickly eradicate pain and is even reported to be effective killing the streptococcus bacteria.

Liquids
- Drinking warm liquids, especially with added honey helps coat the throat and provide comfort.

Section IV

Baselines, Conversions
And
Definitions

Vital Signs

It is important to know what "normal" looks like so that you can identify abnormal. Below is a list of "baseline readings". Use this list as a guideline for identifying a potential problem.

Temperature

There are two kinds of thermometer scales: Centigrade (C.) and Fahrenheit (F.) Either can be used to measure a person's temperature. Here is how they compare:

Fahrenheit	Centigrade
98.6° F is normal	37° C is normal
Below 95° F is too low	Below 35° C is too low
99° to 102° F is some fever	37° to 39° C is some fever
Above 102° F is a high fever	Above 39° C is a high fever

Pulse or Heartbeat

For a person at rest:

ADULTS	60 to 80 beats per minute is normal.
CHILDREN	80 to 100 beats per minute is normal.
BABIES	100 to 140 beats per minute is normal.
NEWBORNS	120 to 160 beats per minute is normal.

* For each degree Centigrade (C.) of fever, the heartbeat usually increases about 20 beats per minute.

Respiration

For a person at rest:

ADULTS AND OLDER CHILDREN	12 to 20 breaths per minute
CHILDREN	up to 30 breaths per minute
BABIES	up to 40 breaths per minute
NEWBORNS	30 to 60 breaths per minute

* More than 40 shallow breaths a minute usually indicates pneumonia.

Blood Pressure

For a person at rest:
120/80 is normal, but this varies a lot.

- A blood pressure monitor is required equipment to accurately measure blood pressure.
- If the second reading (when the sound disappears when listening on a stethoscope) is over 100 this is a danger sign of high blood pressure.

Conversion Chart

1 Kilogram = 2.2 pounds

5 cc = 1 teaspoon

1 quart is slightly less than 1 liter

2 cups = 1 pint

4 cups = 1 quart

Definitions

IV – Intravenous (in the vein)

IM – Intramuscular (in the muscle)

SQ – Subcutaneous (under the skin)

OTC – Over the counter

Section V

Shopping Lists

Resources

Shopping Lists

Personal Protection Equipment

- Nitrile (or latex) Gloves (in your size and one size up)
- Surgical Masks
- Surgical Masks with Face Shields

Bandaging

- Clean or sterile 4x4 gauze sponges
- Gauze rolls
- Vaseline Dressings
- Co-flex (cohesive bandages-stick to themselves)
- Elastic bandages
- Band aids
- Butterfly bandages
- Surgical tape
- Hydrogen Peroxide
- EMT Shears
- Antibiotic ointment (Neosporin, bag balm)
- Petroleum Jelly

Pharmaceuticals (OTC)

- Tylenol (Adult and Children)
- Ibuprofen (Adult and Children)
- Aspirin
- Benadryl
- Robitussin DM Cough Syrup or its generic equivalent
- Loperamide 2mg (for diarrhea and vomiting)
- Meclizine 25mg (for nausea and vomiting)
- Chloroquine (for malaria)

- Primatene Mist (no longer available after 12/11)
- Cough Drops
- Stool Softeners
- Enemas
- Eye drops
- Betadine
- Epsom's Salts
- Alcohol

Antibiotics

- **Amoxicillin** (Pneumonia, Typhoid fever)
- **Ampicillin** (Typhoid fever)
- **Azithromycin** (Pneumonia, Pertussis, Typhoid fever)
- **Chloramphenicol** (Cholera, Typhus, Typhoid fever)
- **Ciprofloxacin** (Bubonic Plague, Typhoid fever)
- **Clarithromycin** (Pertussis)
- **Clindamycin** (Tetanus)
- **Cotrimoxazole** (Cholera)
- **Erythromycin** (Cholera, Pneaumonia, Pertussis, Tetanus)
- **Furazolidone** (Cholera)
- **Metronidazole** (Tetanus)
- **Penicillin** (Tetanus)
- **Streptomycin** (Bubonic Plague, TB)
- **Tetracycline/Doxycycline** (Bubonic Plague, Cholera, Pneumonia, Typhus)
- **Trimethoprin-sulfamethoxazole** (Pertussis, Typhoid fever)

Doctor's Choice
- **Amoxicillin (Pneumonia)**
- **Doxycycline (Cholera)**
- **Erythromycin (if allergic to penicillin) (Scarlet Fever)**
- **Furazolidone (Cholera)**
- **Penicillin (Scarlet Fever)**
- **Tetracycline (Bubonic Plague, Cholera, Pneumonia, Typhus)**

Vitamins/Supplements

- Prenatal vitamins
- Multi-vitamins (both adult and child)
- Potassium Chloride (for Oral Rehydration Therapy)
- Emergen-C

Household Chemicals

- Chlorine Bleach
- Pool Shock (disinfectant – indefinite shelf life)

Miscellaneous

- Bulb syringe
- RescueVac (for suctioning vomit or phlegm)
- Hot water bottle (for comfort and enemas)
- Baby bottles
- Sports bottles
- Drinking straws
- Notebooks
- Teakettle
- Thermometers
- Blood pressure cuff/monitor
- Humidifier
- Plastic garbage bags
- Zip-loc bags
- Syringe without needle (for dispensing medication)
- Medicine dispenser

Recommended Reading

Where there is no Doctor
David Werner, Jane Maxwell, Carol Thuman

Where there is no Dentist
Murray Dickson

A Book for Midwives
Susan Klein, Suellen Miller, Fiona Thomson

The Bird Flu Preparedness Planner
Grattan Woodson, MD

www.armageddonmedicine.net

www.survivalblog.com

www.paratusfamilia.com

Sources

All of the information in this book, with the exception of the sections entitled "The Doctor Says" was derived from the various sources listed below:

Bubonic Plague
- Wikipedia, free encyclopedia

Chickenpox
- Wikipedia, free encyclopedia
- A.D.A.M.

Cholera
- Wikipedia, free encyclopedia
- Centers for Disease Control and Prevention

Dengue Fever
- Where there is no doctor

Hantavirus
- Centers for Disease Control and Prevention
- A.D.A.M.

Head Lice
- Wikipedia, free encyclopedia
- Safe Natural Cures

Malaria
- Where there is no doctor

Measles
- Wikipedia, free encyclopedia

Mumps
- Wikipedia, free encyclopedia

Pneumonia
- Wikipedia, free encyclopedia

Pertussis
- Wikipedia, free encyclopedia

Radiation Poisoning
- eHow.com
- Wikipedia, free encyclopedia

Rubella
- Wikipedia, free encyclopedia

Scarlet Fever
- Wikipedia, free encyclopedia

Smallpox
- Wikipedia, free encyclopedia
- Centers for Disease Control and Prevention
- WebMD

Starvation
- Wikipedia, free encyclopedia
- Gale Encyclopedia of Medicine

Tetanus
- Wikipedia, free encyclopedia
- Mayo Clinic
- Where there is no doctor
- A.D.A.M.

Tuberculosis
- Centers for Disease Control and Prevention

Typhoid Fever
- Wikipedia, free encyclopedia

Typhus
- Wikipedia, free encyclopedia
- A.D.A.M.

Made in the USA
Lexington, KY
01 September 2013